Yoga and the Jesus Prayer

First published by O-Books, 2010
O Books is an imprint of John Hunt Publishing Ltd., The Bothy, Deershot Lodge, Park Lane, Ropley, Hants, SO24 0BE, UK
office1@o-books.net
www.o-books.com

Distribution in:

UK and Europe
Orca Book Services Ltd

Home trade orders
tradeorders@orcabookservices.co.uk
Tel: 01235 465521 Fax: 01235 465555

Export orders
exportorders@orcabookservices.co.uk
Tel: 01235 465516 or 01235 465517
Fax: 01235 465555

USA and Canada
NBN
custserv@nbnbooks.com
Tel: 1 800 462 6420 Fax: 1 800 338 4550

Australia and New Zealand
Brumby Books
sales@brumbybooks.com.au
Tel: 61 3 9761 5535 Fax: 61 3 9761 7095

Far East (offices in Singapore, Thailand, Hong Kong, Taiwan)
Pansing Distribution Pte Ltd
kemal@pansing.com
Tel: 65 6319 9939 Fax: 65 6462 5761

South Africa
Stephan Phillips (pty) Ltd
Email: orders@stephanphillips.com
Tel: 27 21 4489839 Telefax: 27 21 4479879

ISBN: 978 1 84694 285 3

Design: Stuart Davies

A CIP catalogue record for this book is available from the British Library.

Printed in the UK by CPI Antony Rowe
Printed in the USA by Offset Paperback Mfrs, Inc

Yoga and the Jesus Prayer

Thomas Matus

Thomas Matus

BOOKS

Winchester, UK
Washington, USA

CONTENTS

Preface

by Joseph Campbell
(from a personal letter to the author)

Honolulu, Hawaii
April 20, 1985

I am now reading your *Yoga and the Jesus Prayer Tradition* with what I might even call excitement, learning a new vocabulary and discovering new meanings in terms long known to me but otherwise understood. You are kind to have sent me this precious little book, which has already become my guide to a new order of realizations.

The meeting, last month, with you and Brother David was already a clue to me of something going on in your Big Sur Hermitage with which I would do well to become acquainted, and I am now delighted to have received this confirmation of my expectation. Paulist Press, some years ago, advertised a great series of Occidental mystical writings to be published, of which I have been receiving the volumes, one by one, as they have appeared. What I missed was a comprehensive introduction, and that is what you have now given me.

Next year, I shall again be conducting at Esalen a seminar with Al Huang, and I hope to be able to visit and have another talk with you at that time. Meanwhile, my heartfelt thanks.

Sincerely, Joseph Campbell

Other words of praise for the 1984 edition of *Yoga and the Jesus Prayer Tradition*

In the Christian tradition the Body of Christ has had a threefold meaning: Jesus Christ, the Church, and the Eucharist. As a result of a genuine fecundation with the Tantric tradition, Thomas Matus reminds us that it also means the Body of Man. This is a pioneer work in the right direction.

— Raimon Panikkar, author of *The Vedic Experience: Mantramanjari* and *The Cosmotheandric Experience*.

This is an unusual book, bringing together two traditions, that of Eastern Orthodoxy and that of Hindu and Buddhist Tantra, which as far as I know have never been related before. Beneath the obvious differences of conceptual framework the author discovers a remarkable similarity of experience... [Thomas Matus] has given one of the best expositions of the essential meaning of Tantra that I know, and for this alone his work is of great value. But he also shows how the Tantra can be related to Christian experience.

— Bede Griffiths, author of *The Marriage of East and West* and *The Golden String*.

An extraordinary work... The book informs and it inspires us to pause and ponder prayerfully, often in awe at what is being laid before us. Thomas Matus is especially good at cross-cultural spiritual correlations. He neatly relates or connects the physical and psychic ways by which some of us attempt to enter, or begin to enter, the mystery we call God.

— Anthony Wilhelm, author of the Catholic best-seller *Christ Among Us*.

Also by Thomas Matus

Ashram Diary: In India With Bede Griffiths
(O Books, 2009)

Bede Griffiths Essential Writings

Duo concertante
(with Anna M. Pinnizzotto)

Nazarena, an American Anchoress

Chapter I

The Way of Integration

Bede Griffiths said, "There may be another way, but integration of flesh and spirit is Christ's way for us today."

Readers of my *Ashram Diary* (O Books, 2009) will find this phrase on page 60; elsewhere in the book I reflect on the theme of integration through the practice of yoga, which lies at the center of my personal experiment. In September, 1958, I was initiated into a practice that Paramahansa Yogananda, in his *Autobiography of a Yogi*, called Kriya Yoga; the ceremony was guided by his disciples Bhaktananda and Mokshananda. I was eighteen at the time and a sophomore at Occidental College in Los Angeles, a forty-minute walk from Yogananda's monastic center on Mount Washington.

Kriya Yoga is a form of meditation, rooted in the Vedas of Hinduism, as well as in Hindu and Buddhist Tantras or esoteric texts. My own practice of it, my experimentation with the polarities of flesh and spirit, evolved into an experiment in faith. Yogananda, through his yoga technique, was for me a 'guru unto Christ'; his own vision of Jesus suggested an understanding of the universe, both material and spiritual, as a 'mystical body' animated by what Yogananda called 'the Christ consciousness'. Then one day (Friday, June 24, 1960, at about 8:30 in the evening) I realized that I had another guru, the church of Saint Francis, Brother Lawrence, John of the Cross, and the other Christian mystics whom Yogananda mentioned in his writings. I began that evening's meditation as a disciple of Yogananda and a believer in the reincarnation of souls; in an instant, in which I seemed to touch eternity, I was a Catholic and a believer in the resurrection of the flesh. Of course, my reading and study of mystical literature, including a couple of books by the Trappist monk and poet, Thomas Merton, had affected my views and aspirations, but these readings were in no way a gradual preparation for conversion. One minute I was one person; the next I was another.

The suddenness of this turning in faith to Catholic Christianity did not immediately favor my personal integration. The Catholicism I began to study in autobiographical 'convert stories' and apologetic expositions of the faith for adult readers drove a wedge within me between flesh and spirit. The liberal, even leftist ideas I had absorbed from my parents, especially from my mother and her sister, seemed incompatible with the unquestionable certainties of faith and morals in a church that had not yet celebrated its Second Vatican Council. Yet this same church, rock-solid and seamless, had a prophet for a pope, a man more unique than rare, John XXIII. Not only was he what Catholics piously call 'the holy father'; he was truly holy, a living saint and a loving father. Some Catholic converts, like Merton himself and Dorothy Day, made me feel I was in good company in the Catholic Church, in spite of the cognitive dissonance between my instinctive liberalism and what seemed to be the church's immutable doctrines.

Converts buy the 'whole package'; we cannot discern the degrees of truth and certitude as 'cradle Catholics' do. So I felt I had to adopt the most conservative and rigid views I found in the books I read for my instruction, views that Thomas Merton espoused as a fresh convert and expressed in his earlier writings, like the autobiography *The Seven Storey Mountain* (published in England as *Elected Silence*). As literature, this is the best thing Merton wrote, and yet it is a terrible book, so harshly unfair to other faiths and to Merton's own youthful *joie de vivre* that, had I read it while still a member of Yogananda's Self-Realization Fellowship, I might never have become a Catholic. What I did read was *Seeds of Contemplation*, whose publisher made him edit out his contemptuous words about Buddhist *nirvāṇa* and Sufi mysticism for the second printing of the book. I also read *The Sign of Jonas*, which was a deeply sincere narrative of Merton's monastic and priestly initiation; I could relate to what he said there, and his joy at becoming a monk buoyed my hopes of joining Yogananda's disciples in their monastic community.

Having become a Catholic, the solution to my personal dilemma was paradoxical: still struggling with the apparent incompatibility of my liberal ideas with integral Catholicism, I entered the newly-founded Immaculate Heart Hermitage of the Camaldolese, an order that has roots in Benedictine monasticism, but which, for its American foundation, presented itself almost exclusively as an order of hermits. California's New Camaldoli was set into the Santa Lucia Mountains south of the Big Sur coast. There I was confronted with one of the most splendid views on earth: a meandering, rocky coastline and the vast Pacific Ocean, open sea that extended halfway around the earth to the Antarctic. But there was no view at all from the windows of the hexagonal cottages that were the hermits' cells; they looked out on a small garden, circumscribed by a tall, board fence. I thought: sensory deprivation is the yoga of the American Camaldolese hermits.

To allay my convert scruples, I sought out a conservative priest who had transferred to the Camaldolese from the Cistercians of the Strict Observance (they, in his opinion, were not strict enough). He let me go to confession every day, until the novice master ordered me not to. But an Italian monk from Camaldoli in Tuscany and a Jesuit from India showed me, in their way of life and in something implicit in what they said, that being a Catholic and a Camaldolese monk could lead me to a center whose circumference was everywhere, an indivisible point that embraced all humanity and the entire universe.

I still had battle lines drawn through the field of soul and flesh. I was fighting on both sides, against and with my flesh, against and with the thoughts of my soul. I was like Arjuna in the first chapter of the *Bhagavad-Gītā*, standing with his charioteer, Krishna, between the two armies. At times my yoga seemed to be that of this reluctant warrior: the yoga of despair. Learning to meditate with the Bible, I heard my own voice in the last verse of Psalm 88: "My only companion is the darkness."

Thank goodness I heard not only the voice of despair; I heard an inner voice that suggested I should resume practicing yoga, which Yogananda and his gurus called 'a science of the soul' as universal as mathematics and hence compatible with religious devotion of every kind. You can still be a Catholic, the voice told me, and be a Kriya Yogi. Strange to say, my over-sensitized conscience did not allow me to dwell on the disobedience that practicing yoga in an enclosed Catholic order perhaps implied. A hint from the American novice master and half a word from the gentle Italian monk, Aliprando, freed me from this scruple.

A further reinforcement of my choice to be both a Catholic and a yogi came from the Indian Jesuit, Pedro. He invited me to his cell, where he was living in complete reclusion, and showed me the prayer corner at the head of his bed. He had a large image of the Sacred Heart of Jesus joined by images of the Virgin Mary and Aloysius Gonzaga, the patron saint of purity; beneath these images was a photograph of Yogananda. Pedro asked me to demonstrate Kriya Yoga to him, and so I did. Later I found the Italian translation of Yogananda's autobiography on Aliprando's bookshelf; he said he had read it but made no further comment. Thus even the Camaldolese hermits provided me with positive reinforcement of what my liberal mind-set permitted and the inner voice commanded.

When I had been at New Camaldoli for five years, the monks voted me into perpetual vows and sent me and three others to Rome for further studies. My three brothers eventually left the order, and I stayed in Italy, mostly at the mountain monastery attached to the Holy Hermitage of Camaldoli. Living as a 'cenobite' (a community monk) was a healing experience, in a way even more demanding than living as a hermit in a cell at New Camaldoli. After studying theology in Rome, I asked permission to write a doctoral dissertation on yoga, interpreting it as a way into the mystical body of Christ. I also wanted to read the Tantras as sources for what Yogananda called Kriya Yoga, in order to answer some personal questions that Yogananda's printed lessons did not. My Italian superiors let me live outside the order and take a Ph.D. at Fordham University in New York. After returning to the monastery, I had the dissertation published by Paulist Press in 1984, with the title, *Yoga and the Jesus Prayer Tradition: An Experiment in Faith.* This book contains the substance of it, and while revising it a quarter-century later, I have added some personal narrative of my journey with monks, hermits, and lay people, women and men, Christians, Hindus, and Buddhists, on the way to the integration of flesh and spirit, the real purpose of yoga.

The Search for Religious Identity

The final years of the twentieth century marked a time of searching for values, both new and old. The overconfidence of industrial society began to give way to a profound, collective insecurity; individuals often tried to remedy this insecurity by grasping at some form of religious identity. If I can understand myself in terms of an absolute, eternal system of which I am a part, the reasoning goes, nothing can ultimately harm me.

The search for religious identity and for the subjective certitude that goes with it is part of human nature and hence in itself is positive and often necessary for maintaining one's sanity. But the search for religious identity is not the same thing as the spiritual search. Being aware of one's religious roots is comforting, but it is not identical either with faith or with the experience of God. Faith, when it is authentic, takes me beyond security into a realm where peace may indeed be found, but only in an unmoored drifting into the vast sea of reality.

I cast the anchor of my life down, and I let its line run deep into the unfathomable God on whose bosom I float. In this situation, two certitudes reassure me: the one, that it is not madness to be afloat in God, and the other, that I am not alone on this sea.

The search that led me to the Catholic faith at the beginning of my adult life brought me into contact with the doctrines and spiritual disciplines of Hinduism and Buddhism. Since I cannot undo this search without undoing my faith, I cannot live my Christian identity except as a man who came to be a Christian and a monk by reading Hindu scriptures and practicing yoga.

After several years of searching and experimenting in faith, I went looking for a spiritual way native to Christianity that would point me in the same direction I had taken, perhaps without knowing it, when I started my journey with yoga. I found that Christian way in hesychasm. Hesychasm (from the Greek word *hēsychia*, meaning 'quiet' or 'the silent life') is a tradition that developed in the Eastern Church, growing out of the experience and doctrines of the fourth-century and later church teachers who wrote in Greek. Hesychasm was refined as a theology and a way of life in the monastic centers of Mount Sinai, Constantinople, and Athos, and later in Russia and other Eastern European countries. A great hesychast of the twentieth century was the Russian monk Silouan of Mount Athos (1866-1938).

Hesychasm gave me a standard or paradigm with which to evaluate yoga as a spiritual discipline. Yoga, which arose outside Christianity, and hesychasm, which is thoroughly Christian, must have something in common, and this something can be found in the fact that both respond to certain needs of the human person, whose spiritual dynamism found expression in these two ways, among others. We are dealing, then, with a comparison, which immediately raises problems, given the evident differences between hesychasm and yoga.

Mysticism and Eastern Christianity

Some historians and philosophers of religion have made much of the distinction between 'mystical' and 'prophetic' religions, placing in the latter category faiths such as Judaism, Christianity, and Islam, sometimes adding to them Mazdaism (the teaching of Persia's prophet Zarathusthra).[1] Prophetic faiths are 'religions of the word'; they affirm that God, in his [2] sovereignty and otherness, sends his word from on high, a word that judges and even accuses the people, calling them to a change of life in submission to God's will. The great religions of India and the Far East, such as Hinduism, Buddhism, and Taoism, are 'mystical'; in other words, they teach that salvation, liberation, or illumination is an experience of unity beyond all possible conceptualization and expression, an experience that comes from within and that can be reached only by a return to one's center. The West, too, has known mystical religions, especially during the Hellenistic period, before and after the birth of Jesus, when Asian religious influences spread throughout the Roman empire.

One of these influences was Christianity itself,[3] which remains, in many respects, an Asian religion. Although Peter and Paul went west on their Apostolic journeys, other disciples headed for Syria and Persia. According to unbroken oral tradition, Thomas the apostle reached India before Peter arrived in Rome. The first great phase of intellectual, liturgical, and artistic development in the church took place in the Eastern Mediterranean and in Asia.[4] Hence even as a cultural phenomenon, the Christian community is at home in the East as much as in the West, and since its destiny is to be at home everywhere, the inculturation of the gospel will continue to the end of time.

Although its existence is often ignored by those engaged in the East-West dialogue, the Christian East has a distinctive role to play in the meeting of Christianity with the great spiritual traditions of Asia. For many reasons, aside from geographical proximity, the Eastern Church offers Christians a way to approach Asian religious cultures as it were on their home ground.

Many of those who identify the gospel of Christ with Western culture also tend to ignore or deny its mystical dimension. But this idea of an utterly prophetic, non-mystical Christianity of the sovereign word finds little support in Christian history. The gospel faith did indeed spring from a prophetic religion, Judaism, because Jesus was both a Jew and a prophet. But for those who see him as the Word made flesh, he transcends the limits of his own and all other religions. His humanity saves us; the divine incarnate divinizes all human nature. In him we inherit, not a religion or a culture, but God's own life. This is why Christianity cannot confine itself to the categories of prophetic or mystical religion, nor to any culture, Western or Eastern.

Eastern Christianity is often identified with what is called the 'Byzantine' or 'Greek' church. This church is found today largely in Greece, Russia and other Slavic countries, the Near East, Romania (which is, linguistically and culturally, a Latin nation), and North and South America. Other Eastern Christian traditions are the Coptic (Egypt and Ethiopia), the Syrian (Lebanon, Iraq, Iran, and India), and the Armenian (Armenia and the Americas). Although the majority of Byzantine-rite Christians are now in Europe and the Americas, the origins of their liturgy, theology, and spirituality are Asian no less than Greek or Slavic. Many of the early Christian writers who wrote in

Greek lived in Asia Minor, where they came into contact with various ancient cultures of the East.

The chief mystical expression of Eastern Christianity is hesychasm. This contemplative ideal and way of life is deeply rooted in the earliest Christian teachings, especially those of the writers called 'the Cappadocians', that is, Basil the Great, his brother Gregory of Nyssa, and their friend Gregory Nazianzen. Hesychasm reached its full flowering after the eleventh century on Mount Athos, the peninsular monastic republic on Greek soil southwest of Constantinople, modern Istanbul; its fullest theological expression is in the writings of the fourteenth-century bishop and contemplative, Gregory Palamas.

Against their accusers, Palamas defended the monks on Athos who practiced and taught the hesychastic method of prayer (also called 'the Jesus prayer'). His theological writings placed this method within the orthodox doctrinal framework of the church, and he found that hesychasm was implicit in the teachings and experience of early and medieval Christian writers like Symeon the New Theologian.

Saint Symeon (949-1022) is considered by many to be both the greatest medieval mystic of the Eastern Church and a father of hesychasm. He is today one of the saints whose writings are most widely read on Mount Athos and in other monastic centers. Already in the fourteenth century, a text called "Three Methods of Attention and Prayer" had been attributed to Symeon; this short work seems to be the first to describe the physical procedure, often compared to yoga techniques, which some hesychasts practiced as an aid to mental concentration. However, a careful reading of this text in the light of Symeon's authentic writings shows that he cannot have been its author.

Still, Symeon's conception of the mystical life is the same as that which underlies both the practice of hesychasm and Gregory Palamas' doctrinal defense of it. It is not necessary to claim that any particular method originated with Symeon; he is certainly a bridge between the early teachers of the Eastern Church (the Cappadocians, Maximus the Confessor, and others) and the hesychasts of later centuries. It is not by chance that revivals of hesychastic prayer in recent years have been stimulated and nourished by renewed contact with the writings of Symeon the New Theologian. It is in this sense that we are taking his experience as an example of hesychastic spirituality.

The text called "Three Methods of Attention and Prayer" has, as I said, often been considered a manual of 'Christian yoga' because it teaches the contemplative to link the invocation of the name of Jesus with awareness of heart and breath rhythms. However, this similarity is largely superficial. Physical procedures are but the skin of yoga; its sinews and skeleton are mental exercises that lead to the transformation of consciousness. But the soul of yoga is a vision of light that is one, pure, undivided, and beyond all movement and change. One can see how similar or dissimilar yoga and hesychasm really are, only by comparing the highest spiritual experience proper to each.

Christian Meanings of Yoga

Comparing yogic and hesychastic experience is itself a fascinating task, as well as a difficult one. But here we shall go one step further and use the insights gained by comparing and contrasting them as a first step toward answering a question many people are asking today: can the practice of yoga (or, if you wish, zen meditation) lead to an experience that is truly Christian?

This question has nothing to do with syncretism; I personally have no interest in the attempt to blend Christianity with Hinduism or Buddhism into some kind of higher synthesis. Nor do I see any need to adopt the outward trappings of an Asian culture (clothing, diet, etc.) along with its spiritual disciplines. What is at issue for me is the use of yoga as an aid to dedicating my whole being to Christ and in fulfilling Christ's law of loving service to my neighbor.

There are basically two kinds of Christian seekers who turn to yoga. The first are those who feel something is missing in their inner life that cannot be found in the Christianity they know and practice. They especially feel the need of a definite, concrete 'technique' or method of spiritual training, something they can do that will give guaranteed results. Then there are other persons (and these, it seems, are becoming more and more numerous) who undergo a sudden and unexpected spiritual crisis that manifests itself outwardly in many strange ways: electric currents seem to course through the body; lightning explodes in the brain, and they are overwhelmed by a force that is at the same time alien and familiar, a source both of pain and an obscure sense of fulfillment. Then they discover that such an experience is described in books on yoga as 'the awakening of *kuṇḍalinī*', and so they start practicing yoga.

Both kinds of seekers understand that, as a practical method (apart from the metaphysical and theological systems of Hinduism and Buddhism), yoga is no more incompatible with Christianity than is a taste for exotic foods or unconventional attire. But this understanding, that there is nothing necessarily wrong or unorthodox about the adoption of yogic means to the Christian end, does not answer the question why they adopted yoga in the first place.

Maybe this is a useless question. Maybe the practice of yoga, even if it is no more immoral or heterodox than odd tastes in food or clothing, is still only part of the vanity of this world, only one more burden on a soul that really needs to fly in freedom toward God, unburdened by any other 'yoke' than that of Jesus.[5]

I myself have nurtured these doubts. I have felt that yoga is indeed vanity, the burdensome yoke of an 'old law', which cannot save, if it is nothing but 'technique'. But then I discovered that many Hindu and Buddhist writers, even in ancient times, also saw the need to abandon techniques, but, having done so, they still practiced yoga. Maybe, I thought, there is something more to yoga than what is sometimes peddled under that name in the West.

So yoga is not just 'techniques'. What, then, is it?

Yoga has assumed many different forms during the several thousand years it has been practiced; it is impossible to define it simply and exactly. It grew into a high art within the context of Indian religious culture, but there have been forms of spiritual discipline outside India (shamanism, Christian monasticism, sufism, etc.) that resemble yoga in some way. Following the missionary expanse of Buddhism, elements of yoga spread throughout Asia, and in the twentieth century, Yogananda and others have taught yoga in the West, suggesting new ways of adapting its age-old principles and practices to non-Asian cultures.

In the West, what yoga has become, more than anything else, is a symbol of the vocation to an interior, spiritual life and a symbol of the universality of this vocation. Yoga is a skill, an art, and as such it is much better characterized as 'wisdom' than as 'science'.

Everyone knows what music is, and yet there are innumerable forms and styles of music. In the same way, the art of yoga, impossible to define exactly, embraces countless methods and 'styles' in its practical application.

The term 'tantric yoga' refers to those forms of yoga that were developed and applied in certain schools of Buddhism and Hinduism, beginning in the first centuries of the common era. Tantrism is so called because its principal scriptural authority is the body of anonymous writings called Tantras. A Tantra is a treatise or elaboration of oral religious teachings. These texts were believed to supersede the more ancient scriptures, the Vedas and Upanishads. Tantric apologetics sometimes claimed a primeval origin for the Tantras; they were the 'eternal word' adapted to humanity living in a 'dark age'.

Tantrism is often identified with Shaktism, the devotion to the *śakti*, 'power' or 'energy' personified as a Divine Mother. The yoga of Hindu Tantrism is also referred to as '*kuṇḍalinī yoga*'. The term *kuṇḍalinī* means 'coiled' or 'serpentine' and describes the form of *śakti* residing in the human body as a potential force coiled like a serpent at the base of the body's vertical axis. The practice of yoga aims at 'awakening' and 'uncoiling' the *kuṇḍalinī-śakti* and making it rise to the 'abode of God' at the crown of the head. It is important to remember that not all Hindu Tantrism can be called Shaktism, and the awakening of the inner *śakti* is not the sole aim of tantric yoga. Both yoga and Tantrism are historically complex, and it is misleading to oversimplify them.

Experience and Faith

By entering into the spirituality of the Eastern Orthodox Church, I discovered that I could 'turn to the East' and draw nearer to the religious psychology of India, where yoga was born, while still affirming my Christian identity. But why did I focus on tantric yoga?

I did not make this choice arbitrarily. Of all the historical schools of yoga, Tantrism seems to imply a view of human existence closer to a Christian 'incarnate' view than that of any other yogic school. Tantric writers often have a more holistic understanding of human nature than does, for example, the legendary author of the *Yoga Sūtras*, Patañjali. Above all, the vocabulary of symbols in which tantric texts are couched has much in common with the way Symeon the New Theologian and those who followed him talked about their mystical experience. But can mystical experience itself be compared?

It is not really my purpose to answer this question here. I am convinced that there is a great variety in mysticism and among mystics; experiences that are apparently similar are not necessarily identical, and experiences had outside the visible confines of Christianity, although they may appear very different from those of a Saint Symeon, may in fact, by the inscrutable action of grace, be a true mystical experience of the God whom I seek in Christ. So my purpose in comparing the way Symeon and the yogis speak about their respective experiences is not simply to see where they agree or disagree. What ultimately interests me is how the yogic discipline and its experiential fruits can be interiorized in terms of the Christian faith I embraced, after my initiation into Kriya Yoga.

What is experience? One of the greatest teachers I met in Rome, the monk Cipriano Vagaggini, defined it as the direct, non-conceptual knowledge of a present reality.[6] When Vagaggini said that experience is non-conceptual, he did not mean that it cannot be intellectual. The intellect, he explained, also has an obscure, concomitant experience of its own activity and of the self as the ground of that activity. On a human plane, experience of anything other than myself comes about by 'connaturality'; that is, I know the other through the other's value for myself, through my attraction to, or repulsion from, the other. This connaturality or, in other words, my subjective disposition as knower in relation to the known, is the medium of experiential knowledge, much as the idea or formal concept in the mind is the medium of abstract, intellectual knowledge.

What impressed me most in Vagaggini's teaching, was his repeated affirmation that experience involves the total person, body, mind, and spirit, within the living context of a wider, cosmic totality. The world, the body, and the senses are very much a part of even the most spiritual experience of the self and its activity. All experience points beyond the dichotomies of self and other, of subject and object, because experience really unites the knower to the known and to the universe, which encompasses them both. Thus in every experience, I perceive, if only obliquely, both my being in its totality and my being-in-the-world.

Faith is a way of knowing that points beyond the world, because it is a real, direct contact with God, the absolute origin of the world. Faith also has its kind of experience, which is like no other. The act of faith is above all a grace that transforms mind, heart, and senses, and plunges them into the 'divine darkness', into a 'cloud of unknowing' that is the personal presence of the living God.

In a certain sense, there can be no connaturality between myself and God. On a purely human plane, the relationship of connaturality begins with the self, the subject, who reaches toward, or 'intends', the object, but on the plane of faith, the 'energy' in the act of knowing flows as it were along an elliptical path around two foci, which are the divine and human natures.

My knowledge of God by faith is a consequence of God's knowing me from all eternity. I know because first I am known, and when my knowledge is perfected in love, it will be a genuine 'participation in the divine nature' (cf. II Peter 1:4). This is not a subjective disposition of the knower; it is a divine disposition or 'dispensation' (*oikonomia*), in which God knows each human person in the incarnate Word. It is God's self-knowing that makes God knowable.

The value of experience in the life of faith is at least as great as the value of experience in human life in general. Experience is the culmination and end of faith and of the life that flows from it; experience is what moves me to bear active witness to faith, and it is also a necessary condition for the intellectual understanding of faith, that is, for theology.

The experience of faith takes place on three levels: (1) there is self-knowledge, that is, the knowledge of my whole person in relationship with God; (2) there is the knowledge of God by the connaturality of grace, that is, by my real participation in the divine nature; and (3) there is the participation of my senses, emotions, and imagination in the faith-experience and hence a real transformation of the body. These three levels are always present; however, one may predominate over the others in a given experience. I may also know God in other ways: for example, by an intellectual, conceptual knowledge of God, or theological knowledge, although this way of knowing is inferior to mystical experience, toward which theological thinking must always tend.

I seek to understand my experience in accord with the objective content of the faith. In other words, I submit my experience to the judgment and guidance of spiritual authority (Sacred Scripture and the tradition of the church, the discernment of my spiritual director, etc.), and I examine myself in the light of the Sermon on the Mount (Matthew, chapters 5-7) and the example of Jesus, to see if my experience is bearing fruit in action, as an authentic sign of the Holy Spirit's grace in me (cf. Galatians 5:22-23).

I can enjoy an experiential consciousness that even gives me a kind of certitude of the Spirit's presence and operation within my soul. But the consciousness of indwelling Spirit is a kind of certitude that Vagaggini taught me to distinguish carefully from an abstract, philosophical certitude of the intellect as well as from the certitude affirmed by convinced religious believers. This is because faith and the experience and understanding that flow from it are always an act of adoration, a prostration of my total being before the Inaccessible and Unknowable One who yet knows me, enters my soul, and thus turns my unknowing into knowledge, however obscure it may be.

Living by faith, I have learned to live in holy fear of this Loving Darkness, and I fear to love my own pale lights more than God's love. I live in the reverential acknowledgment of the chance I may go astray and be deceived, if my mind rebels against the Hidden God. For this reason, my experience, the consciousness of my transformation by the Spirit's intimate presence, needs to be constantly purified. This process of purification involves the dialectic of alternating states, of ups and downs; in fact, the certitude of God's presence often gives way to the experience of God's 'absence'. This happened to Symeon the New Theologian, and it has certainly happened to me.

Experience and the Language of Symbols

Because experience is non-conceptual, it is consequently ineffable. However, all experience points in some way to the structures of our existence as thinking beings embodied in the world. For this reason, I can communicate my experience to another person on the basis of our shared existential context. This communication is accomplished primarily by symbols.[7] Although different writers use different terminologies in their discussion of symbols, most of them distinguish two types of symbolic language: one in which the symbolic term (image, word, etc.) refers to that which is symbolized only or primarily on the basis of an arbitrary convention (e.g., traffic lights), and another in which the symbol is intrinsically related to the reality signified. This latter category (which we may call 'real symbols' as opposed to 'conventional symbols') is what I use to communicate my experience to another person. A 'real symbol' is one whose very being is a manifestation of, and a participation in, another reality. It is an image, an 'icon', which makes present and gives what it signifies. But the reality manifested in the symbol still remains in some way hidden, not so much because the symbol is inadequate or dissimilar, but because the reality has meaning that exceeds any possibility of communication: it is in some way an unknowable mystery.

All experience involves my entire being; likewise, a symbol is a form of communication that expresses my whole being and addresses the whole being of those with whom I communicate. For this reason, symbolic discourse is not subjective or arbitrary, but is grounded in the same reality as experience: in the structures of the human psyche and our shared being-in-the-world. Every symbol is rooted in the totality of human existence, even before it is given concrete expression in art, poetry, or ritual.

The analytical psychologist Carl Jung practiced a kind of 'archeology' of symbols, by digging into what he called the 'collective unconscious' present in the individual psyche, whose 'archetypes' are an inborn potentiality for generating certain kinds of symbols. The archetypes of the collective unconscious are unknowable in themselves, but their existence is deduced from the emergence of identical or similar symbols in widely separated cultural contexts or in the dreams and fantasies of different individuals. Hence, no symbol has ever been created out of nothing by some individual or by a socio-cultural group; instead, it ultimately proceeds from the totality of our existence as a race, and its prehistory begins with the origin of humanity.[8]

Analytical psychologists emphasize this prehistory of symbols, their rootedness in humanity's collective existence and experience. However, we need an equal emphasis on the forward dynamism of symbols, which reflect not only our primordial past but also our future and our ultimate destiny. As a manifestation of human nature and the structures of our existence, a symbol also reflects and anticipates the process of growth toward final perfection, both individual and collective. Symbols reflect the intrinsic bipolarity of human nature; they manifest the tension between the givenness of our nature and the challenge of our existence, between conceptual and non-conceptual knowing, between our embodiment within the material universe and our intrinsic dynamism toward transcendence in God, etc.

This is why all symbolic discourse has a religious dimension, implicit or explicit. This religious meaning of symbols in general is supported by empirical data that Jung and others have gathered in their study of symbolism in dreams and cultural history.[9] Christian revelation is also rooted in the symbolic language of the human psyche. Christianity is not only, not even primarily, a system of dogmas or conceptualized expressions of faith; it is a universal story, a ritual whose efficacious signs speak to more than just my intellect. Above all it is a personal ideal, an image of what I can and must be. Christianity is first and last the person of Jesus Christ, the Word incarnate who assumed the experiential and symbolic dimensions of human understanding and communication, who reveals God not only in his verbal teaching but in his whole existence and activity as a human being, including his death on a cross. Since I believe that his death has meaning in his resurrection, I can see the same meaning in every symbol and myth of dying-and-rising. Indeed, as I discover Christ in myself, I am able to descry in every symbol, whether it comes from my own or another's dream, or from other myths and religions, a meaning that relates to him.

If I read a specific meaning — the vital significance of the Christ-symbol for me — into tantric symbolism, I do not do so in an arbitrary way, nor with the intention of distorting it within its proper context. I shall try to show, in the following chapter, the great variety that yoga and Tantrism have assumed throughout history; today, Hindus and Buddhists who practice forms of tantric yoga hold widely different understandings of the meaning and end of their practice. They all read their experience in the light of teachings and ideals received by faith from authorities they venerate: sacred writings, the gurus, etc. As a Christian I have done the same.

---

1 Cf. R. C. Zaehner, *Concise Encyclopedia of Living Faiths* (London: Hutchinson, 1977).

2 This is not inclusive language, of course, given that the God of most prophets is in fact personified in masculine terms.

3 Cf. Arnold Toynbee, ed., *The Crucible of Christianity: Judaism, Hellenism, and the Historical Background to the Christian Faith* (New York: World Publishing, 1969).

4 Cf. Nicholas Zernov, *Eastern Christendom: A Study of the Origin and Development of the Eastern Orthodox Church* (New York: Putnam, 1961).

5 Cf. Harvey Cox, *Turning East: The Promise and the Peril of the New Orientalism* (New York: Simon and Schuster, 1977).

6 Cf. Cipriano Vagaggini, "Esperienza," Ermanno Ancilli, ed., *Dizionario enciclopedico di spiritualità*, Vol. I, A-J (Rome: Editrice Studium, 1975), pp. 720-727. Vagaggini was also a strong supporter of Bede Griffiths' life in India, at the ashram of Shantivanam; see my *Ashram Diary* (O Books, 2009).

7 Cf. *Symbolisme et théologie*, Studia Anselmiana 64 (Rome: Editrice Anselmiana, 1974; Alexander Schmemann, *For the Life of the World: Sacraments and Orthodoxy* (Crestwood, N.Y.: St. Vladimir's Seminary Press, 1973); contemporary cognitive philosophers, such as George Lakoff, prefer the term 'metaphor' to 'symbol': cf. George Lakoff and Mark Johnson, *Philosophy in the Flesh: The Embodied Mind and Its Challenge to Western Thought* (New York: Basic Books, 1999).

8 Cf. C. G. Jung, *The Structure and Dynamics of the Psyche*, tr. R. F. C. Hull, The Collected Works of C. G. Jung 8 (Princeton: Princeton U. Press, 1969).

9 Cf. C. G. Jung, ed., *Man and His Symbols* (Garden City, N.Y.: Doubleday, 1964).

Chapter II

Tantric Yoga and the Quest for Perfect Freedom

In the religious history of India, the way of the Tantras is revolutionary; it is a new revelation. The 'old law' of the Vedas no longer speaks to the concrete situation of humankind, striving to emerge from the *kali yuga*, the 'dark age'.[1] Tantrism's newness, its revolutionary character, stands out clearly against the background of both Buddhism and Hindu orthodoxy; the Tantras often claim that their doctrine rises above the conflicting traditions of established religions. At the same time, tantric yoga's roots are deep in the history of ancient India.

Indian history is usually thought to begin with the invasion of the subcontinent by semi-nomadic tribes called Aryas.[2] These tribes, a warlike people with a pastoral economy, spoke a form of Sanskrit; the earliest documents of their religious and social culture are the three most ancient texts (third millennium BCE) in any Indo-European language, the Vedas (*Ṛgveda, Sāmaveda, Yajurveda*; a fourth text, *Atharvaveda*, is of later origin, while containing some ancient verses). Consisting mostly of hymns to the Unique One (*tad ekam*; *ekam sat*) under various names and forms, the Vedas also give clues to the advent of the Aryas in modern India and Pakistan, which the nomads entered probably by way of what is now Afghanistan.

Aryan society was structured in much the same way as that of other, related peoples: Persians, Hittites, early Greeks and Latin-speakers. Religious, military, and economic activities were divided among three hereditary castes: the *brāhmaṇas* (priests), the *kśātriyas* (warriors and nobles), and the *vaiśyas* (property-owners and craftsmen). Below the three *āryan* (= 'noble') castes were the *śūdras*, slaves, often of different origin and skin-color from their masters.

Religious activities, especially sacrifice, were all-important for the Aryas; hence the *brāhmaṇas* or 'brahmins' exercised enormous authority. For this reason, the religion of the Vedas is often called 'Brahmanism'. This was in no sense a 'primitive' religion; it was highly refined in thought and symbolism, and even showed signs of the crisis of ritualism that would later come to a head with the Upanishads and early Buddhism.

Aryan religion and culture were not, however, the sole source of the religious ideas and practices we see in Hinduism today. Many of these derive instead from the great prehistoric civilization that the Aryas found already established in India when they arrived. This is the 'Indus Valley culture' or 'Harappan civilization' (from Harappa, the site of one of its principal cities), whose founding dates back perhaps to the third millennium BCE, when other prehistoric civilizations such as those of Egypt and Sumer flourished. The people of the Indus Valley were in many ways more advanced culturally and technologically than the Aryas, but were no match for them militarily.

As the Aryas became dominant in the Indus Valley and beyond, they allowed the local population to retain most of their own religious practices, provided they accepted the ultimate authority of the castes and the Vedas. The Buddha's rejection of this brahmanical orthodoxy in the sixth century BCE was an early, and for some time successful, attempt to challenge the classical aryan social and religious structures and doctrines. The appearance of the first Tantras (perhaps before 300 CE) represented a re-emergence of pre-aryan religious elements above the surface of Brahmanism and Buddhism; Tantrism then spread as a kind of popular counteroffensive against both the vedic priesthood and the established Buddhist orders.

Yoga itself already represented a non-aryan element in Hinduism.[3] An indication of yoga's ancient origins can be seen in photographs of Harappan artifacts; one sculpture shows a bearded man wearing what seems to be a sacred vestment, seated in an attitude similar to later images of yogis and the Buddha: his eyes are half-open, focused on the tip of his nose, and his face bespeaks a profound inner calm.[4]

Archeological remains of the Harappan or Indus Valley civilization also include a number of seals in steatite or copper that represent a sacred figure seated in a typical yoga posture: the legs are bent so that the soles touch one another, with the heels pressed against the perineum; the arms are extended, and the hands rest on the knees.[5] The figure is adorned with bracelets, breastplate, and a horned headdress; he is surrounded by animals of the forest. Other seals show the same figure seated alone, with or without his ornaments, sometimes in a tree, and often as the object of worship.[6] Although scholars differ in their reading of the symbolism in these seals, it seems probable that the image represents the aboriginal deity later called Rudra or Shiva, the lord of yogis and animals.

All yogis, ascetics, and shamans have common ancestors, men and women who used various physical and psychological exercises in order to transcend cyclic time and to emerge from the common lot of humanity into 'immortality and freedom'.[7] Yoga is unique in its highly developed and refined use of such exercises, and pre-aryan India was the soil in which the seeds of later yoga fell, sank their roots, and grew. The Aryas succeeded in imposing their sacred texts and sacrificial rites on the original population, but the soul of pre-aryan religion ultimately prevailed in the penetration first of yoga, then of Tantrism into every level of Indian society and every school of Hinduism, as well as into Buddhism and other Indian traditions, not excluding Christianity and Islam.

Perhaps the one element in Tantrism that reveals most clearly its archaic origins is the centrality of the Divine Mother.[8] This religion of the Mother has a great number of expressions: she is a deity, an object of worship; she is *śakti*, the 'power' or 'energy' of the male divinity's self-manifestation in the cosmos; she is *kuṇḍalinī*, the 'potential force', at once natural and divine, which abides within the human body and which bears the soul upward toward the realization of its own divinity; she is, for Buddhists, the supernal Wisdom, *prajñā-*

paramitā, which leads every sentient being to the discovery of the being's own buddhahood. The feminine in Tantrism does not supplant the male aspect but rather asserts symbolically the complementarity of the two, even on the spiritual level. This complementarity is at once the image of the divine order in both the cosmos and the divinity itself, and it is the intrinsic condition of each human person.

The Tantras present their 'new' doctrine as meeting our human needs in this dark age.[9] We are incapable of the ascetic rigors of the ancients and are slower in grasping their speculative and mystical insights; the ascent to liberation must now begin on a lower plane. Discarding traditional austerities and official worship, the tantric yogis engaged in disciplines and rites that were indeed acted out externally but that increased in value as they were elevated toward another, more subtle plane, or, in other words, as they were interiorized.[10]

The dialectic between the 'gross' and the 'subtle' dominates all of tantric speculation and practice. This dialectic is also closely connected with the obscure and paradoxical style of many tantric writings.[11] Our principal difficulty in understanding them consists in determining how we are to understand a yogic experience expressed in a given text: whether as 'gross' or 'subtle' or both. In any case, the fundamental intention is always the same: to pass from the gross to the subtle, but then to permeate the gross with the value and meaning of the subtle.

This dialectic of interpenetrating planes of reality is not, of course, original with Tantrism; it is present in all of Indian thought. Some hymns of the *Ṛgveda* already manifest the vedic seers' intense concern with finding the 'within' of things, the one reality deep in the core of all that is. Just as the phenomena are manifold, but reality is one, even so the spirit hidden in the human heart (*ātman*) is one with the universal spirit (*brahman*). This fundamental mystical intuition received many different philosophical interpretations in the course of history. Tantric writers also, when they turn to speculation, occupy a wide range of positions, but their starting point, the fundamental intuition, links them to vedic antecedents.[12]

Another link with both vedic Hinduism and early Buddhism is, of course, the practice of yoga. In fact, it is this practice that effects the interpenetration of the gross and the subtle in both theory and reality. By means of yoga, Tantrism joins iconography to alchemy, breath control to ritualized sex, so that they all become means to a single end, the realization of supreme consciousness, unity, and freedom.[13]

An important example of the equivalence of different means in Tantrism is the identification of yoga exercises with cultic actions. This is done in two ways: by giving psycho-physical practices a ritual meaning and value, and by projecting external ritual objects and actions upon the body, thus moving them to an interior and more subtle plane. Paramahansa Yogananda and his guru, Swami Sri Yukteswar, offer examples of both procedures. In 1920, when Yogananda began his work in the United States, he used the term *yogoda* to label both the yogic methods transmitted to him by his guru and the community for 'world brotherhood' that he hoped to initiate in America. After establishing a residential center in Los Angeles, he reverted to the traditional expression, 'Kriya Yoga'. In Sanskrit, *kriyā* is a generic term for ritual actions and 'Kriya Yoga' in *Yoga Sūtras* 2:1 denotes the last three of the five ascetical precepts (*niyama*), 'fervor', 'study of sacred teachings', and 'surrender to God'. Yukteswar preferred the term *yajña*, which refers to the vedic rites that only a scion of the hereditary priesthood may perform. Both guru and disciple were making the same point: yoga is a true sacrifice, and its practitioners are authentic 'priests', whatever may be their caste or nationality.[14]

These tantric identifications are a further development of the theme of 'interior sacrifice' already present in the Upanishads and based on the ancient 'Hymn of the Cosmic Person' in *Ṛgveda* 10:90. The hymn contemplates an archetypal Body, which grows to fill all space, as the various phenomena of the cosmos are formed from the body's members by means of the primal sacrifice. Many passages in the Upanishads also see yoga practice and the experiences that result from it as valid substitutes for vedic rites.[15] Thus Tantrism maintains continuity with vedic tradition, but it also breaks free of it. Instead of the ancient authorities, there are new texts and the gurus who interpret them; in place of brahmanic ritual there are new forms of initiation, sacrifice, and worship; even the practices of earlier yogis are abandoned in favor of new techniques.

A separate problem is the actual beginning of the tantric movement. Scholars speak vaguely of 'the first centuries of the common era', and opinions differ whether Tantrism first arose in Buddhist circles and from there spread to Hinduism, or vice versa.[16] But the originality of either Hindu or Buddhist Tantras is less important than the fact of mutual influence between the two traditions, influences that accompany the entire history of the tantric movement and that were strongest at the high points of its history. For example, Naropa, one of the founders of the Kagyupa school of Tibetan Tantrism, was born in Bengal (the homeland of Yogananda and his gurus) and in 1026, at the age of eleven, went to Kashmir, "at that time the main seat of Buddhist learning."[17] But Kashmir was also the center of the Trika school of Hindu Tantrism, and in the year 1026 one of Hinduism's greatest minds, Abhinavagupta, was perhaps still alive or had only recently died. It was certainly in places and times such as these that ideas passed back and forth between Buddhists and Hindus, enriching both traditions.[18]

Tantrism's golden age in the tenth to twelfth centuries was followed by its gradual decline during the period of Muslim rule in India and its fall into disfavor under British domination. Because of the decadence of some of its later schools and above all because of Western ideological influences, tantric yoga came to be looked upon as an aberrant and and corrupt form of Hinduism and Buddhism. Nevertheless, its presence can still be seen in popular religious practices, especially the worship of the Divine Mother, and in the vitality of the Kagyupa and other tantric systems of Tibetan Buddhism. Tantrism also lives on in Yogananda's lineage, even though its presence therein is purposely veiled. Hence Tantrism today is more than just a living fossil.

Elements of Tantric Practice

This brief sketch of the historical roots of Tantrism helps us understand the central fact in its history: that the yogis' quest for perfection was not bound to any particular system of dogmas, whether philosophical or religious. The origins of both yoga and Tantrism antedate the Vedas and emerge into subsequent history in opposition or at least juxtaposition to the Vedas. There have been tantric systems in Hinduism and in Buddhism; there have been yogas that aimed at union with a personal God and yogas that aimed only at the highest point of consciousness in each stage of the evolution of spirit.

The relative independence of tantric yoga from the dogma-systems in which it has been practiced justifies the method outlined in the first chapter of this book. Just as those who worship Shiva and those who take refuge in the Buddha read their respective world-views and value-systems into yoga, so having become a Christian I sought to read my faith with all its consequences into my practice and experience of the spiritual method I had received from Yogananda's disciples. The grace of faith was (and is) essential for me; all else is auxiliary. Yoga belongs to the order of means, even though it has its own intrinsic end, which, in the concrete situation, can be made to coincide with my ultimate end as a Christian: loving union with God, through transformation into Christ, by the working of the Holy Spirit who dwells within me. In this sense, a Christian understanding of yoga means consciousness of my end in all the means I employ and in all the experiences I undergo throughout the yogic quest. If this understanding is possible, it is because the many different Hindu and Buddhist understandings were possible and were in fact achieved.

However, tantric yoga is not a mere name without any objective and specific content. Through all the variants in its history, there appear certain constants, especially in its view of human nature and of humanity's evolution. It is the anthropology implicit in Tantrism that will guide our understanding of it.

The great historian of yoga, Mircea Eliade, gives us the following point of departure: "The flesh, the living cosmos, and time are the three fundamental elements of tantric *sādhana*."[19] This point of departure determines the practice of yoga's *sādhana* or quest for perfection. In other words, tantric yoga takes us as we are: carnal, worldly, and temporal. It offers us a goal that is not liberation from the human condition but the realization of freedom in time, the world, and the flesh. It is the interplay and integration of these three elements that carries the yogi forward to the goal. The body, the world, and time define the human condition, but they are also the instruments by which the human condition is to be transcended. This transcending does not eliminate the body, the world, or time; instead, as the yogi draws near to perfection, these three elements cease to constitute either means or impediments to the yogi's freedom. Perfection in tantric yoga is the state of the *jīvanmukta*: one who is 'freed while living', who enjoys the complete liberty of the spirit while still in the flesh. For this reason, the Tantras emphasize the value of the body and of all human experience, including some experiences outside the limits of conventional morality.

The Flesh

In the classical system of the *Yoga Sūtras*, the normal, biological life of the body is an instrument of the soul but also something that must ultimately be discarded. The postures and other bodily disciplines (*āsanas*) are a way of acting and being contrary to the spontaneous tendency of the body. To move and to change is of the body's nature; the *āsanas* keep it immobile. The breath flows continually but irregularly; the breathing exercises (*prāṇāyāma*) aim at regulating and then arresting respiration. The senses are by nature aimed at the outside world; the technique of reversing their spontaneous direction (*pratyāhāra*) 'switches off' the flow of sensory information from without.[20]

Tantric yoga employs similar practices, but with a subtly different emphasis. The human condition of embodiment is regarded as a sacred vow and a gift; the body is precious and indispensable for the attainment of spiritual perfection.[21] Poses or postures enable the body to withstand the intense forces unleashed in mediation; an important hatha yoga text states that the awakening of the inner fire (*kuṇḍalinī*) "bakes the earthenware pot" of the body, so that it will not "dissolve in the waters" of this passing world.[22] The yogi is to control the senses, not just by turning them away from their usual objects, but by allowing sense experience to trigger a state of consciousness in which my mind is expanded into a wider dimension. Kriya Yoga has enabled me to control my breathing, stabilize it, and make it observe a slow and hieratic rhythm, without forcing the lungs to retain the air. Thus the act of breathing has become for me a means for transcending time, as well as the vehicle or support for a wide variety of mental projections and meditations.

The most important element in Tantrism's understanding of the body is its analysis of the body-psyche relationship. Just as there are parts of the body that are more or less necessary for sustaining its life, likewise different points in the human anatomy have different relations to consciousness. My body has both a center and an apex: the heart and the 'thousand-petaled lotus' at or just above the crown of the head; it is a space within which energy moves, following the body's vertical axis.[23] The yogic *sādhana* is both a march toward the center and an upward journey. When I began this quest, I realized how little conscious I was of my own body and how difficult it was to experience the different levels of consciousness that coincide with the 'centers' and 'channels' described in Yogananda's lessons. Only after long practice did I begin to orient myself and move freely within my own bodily space.

I gradually recognized the link between flesh and spirit at certain points within the body. This varying level of consciousness in the body is the consequence of an internal dynamism or force called *prāṇa*. *Prāṇa* is closely linked with the breath, although it is not the same as the air in the lungs or nostrils. The vital force of *prāṇa* passes through a multitude of 'channels' (*nāḍīs*) and is concentrated in various 'centers of consciousness' (*cakras*, literally, 'wheels', also called *padmas* or 'lotuses') located at intervals along the axis of the spinal column. In Hindu Tantrism, *prāṇa* in the body also takes the form of *kuṇḍalinī*, the potential energy of human evolution, imagined as a serpent coiled at the base of the spine.

Although these centers of consciousness are not simply identified with organs of the physical body, they are often associated with the following anatomical points: the base of the spine (the basal center), the genital region (the 'water' center), the navel (the 'fire' center), the heart (the 'air' center), the throat and oral cavity (the 'space' or 'ether' center), the forehead (the frontal or 'third-eye' center), and the crown of the head (the center of the Absolute or the 'thousand-petaled lotus'). Yogis discover intrinsic connections between genital and frontal centers and between navel and throat centers, while all the centers ultimately converge in the 'lotus of the heart'.

My initial perception of the polarities of center and circumference, of base and summit, and of the 'lotuses' or centers of consciousness in the body made me realize that I would not find the still point of the revolving inner universe, nor reach the apex of my spirit, until I had experienced the integration of the inner with the outer, the higher with the lower, or, in other words, *nirvāṇa* within my 'profane' existence as an embodied spirit.

I also needed to clarify in my own mind the subtle-gross dialectic, which is fundamental to the language of the Tantras. This dialectic does not coincide with the distinction between the physical and the spiritual. On the contrary, the spiritual is not always 'subtle' nor is the 'gross' level of reality the same as the physical, in the sense of what is empirically observable. Indian metaphysics has always affirmed the distinction between spirit and matter (schools that do not are exceptions that prove the rule), even in those monistic systems that identify the All with consciousness or the Self (*ātman*), in which case, matter is either pure illusion (as in the Vedanta of Shankara) or the manifestation of consciousness (as in Abhinavagupta's monism). The subtle is not a third entity between spirit and matter but rather a difference of quality in the perception of both material and spiritual reality.

The yogis were not interested in providing a medically accurate description of the physical anatomy. Their attention was focused on the transformation of the body into a fit instrument for the spirit, in order to reach a state of consciousness in which the physical body and the cosmic body, the human spirit and the divine Spirit, were perceived in perfect unity. Meditation on the centers of consciousness in my body, strung like flowers in a garland along the cerebro-genital axis, helped me to realize this rupture of planes, the passage from an experience of the body in its isolation and separateness to the experience of its continuity with the All.

The visualizations of the *cakras* given in tantric texts are excellent examples of the subtle-gross dialectic.[24] Letters, colors, sounds, divine images, etc., are projected upon corresponding points along the spinal axis, leading to the integration of consciousness as expressed in various ways: language, religious devotion, aesthetic experience, or bodily awareness. The yogi's consciousness, thus integrated, drives the release and elevation of the potential energy or *kuṇḍalinī*.

The essential instrument for awakening the inner fire is the body itself. Sounds and colors, 'lotuses' and 'wheels' serve as supports for meditation, until I am aware of the *kuṇḍalinī* dynamic. In the end, the separate centers dissolve. Thus it is of little importance whether there are four, six, or eight *cakras*, since meditation on the various points along the body's axis is only an aid in concentrating on the dynamic movement of the inner fire.[25]

Parallel to the subtle-gross dialectic in the body-psyche relationship is the other important polar symbol in the Tantras: that of the female and the male. 'Realization' in tantric yoga, that is, *sādhana* as both process and goal, is often described in sexual terms, as a relationship between the masculine and the feminine on many different levels: the sexual attraction of two human bodies, the convergence between Nature and Spirit, and the mystical union between the soul and God. Tantric texts, although not always consistent in their use of sexual symbolism, present the relationship between the male and the female as a concrete symbol of the polar dualities in human existence, which the yogi seeks to unify.

The Cosmos

Another fundamental polarity in human consciousness is that between the body and the world of which it is a part, or, in other words, between the microcosm (the human person) and the macrocosm (the universe). Yoga deals with this polarity the way it does with others: it accepts the polar dialectic and interiorizes the symbols that represent the duality of person and universe, to the end of overcoming all duality.

Indian thought from its origins held that the cosmos is reflected in the individual and the individual in the cosmos. The 'Hymn of the Cosmic Person' (*Ṛgveda* 10:90) sees the universe as a giant body, whose members constitute the cosmic components as well as the order of society and whose metabolism and growth are the evolution of all things. This primal human is the 'matter' of the original sacrifice offered by gods and ancestral sages. The Upanishads see the universe as a body and in the body. Within the heart is the seed of all things, the *ātman*; thus the individual is a 'little world', a microcosm. Of course there is nothing exclusively Indian in this symbolism; even contemporary scientists have found reasons for affirming the 'cosmic connection' of the human body.[26]

Tantric yoga offers a practical application of the microcosm-macrocosm connection. The transformation of my human condition as being-in-the-world begins with the awakening of 'cosmic consciousness'.[27] I effect this by means of 'projection' or mental identification of my bodily dimensions with the dimensions of the universe. In meditation I seek to interiorize the planets, stars, and galaxies in relation to the points of consciousness along the body's cerebro-genital axis. My visualizations reflect less the symbolism of the Tantras than the 'space dreams' and images of 'alien contact' that have been part of my inner life since early childhood. Ascribe this imagery to science-fiction novels and cinema if you will, but my experience is what it is, and I have tried to integrate it into my spiritual search.

Tantric texts conceive of the spinal column as Mount Meru, the Hindu Olympus or 'center of the world', about which revolve the sun and the moon. These heavenly bodies are often identified with the two lateral 'channels', the *piṅgalā* and the *iḍā*, alongside the *suṣumnā-nāḍī* at the center of the spinal column. As I practice Kriya Yoga, I direct the flow of *prāṇa* within *iḍā* and *piṅgalā* toward the central channel and thence through the six main centers of consciousness. Yogananda identified these centers with the signs of the zodiac, twelve in number as a result of the left-right polarity of *iḍā* and *piṅgalā*; he taught his disciples to direct the mind, and hence the *prāṇa*, successively to each *cakra* in the ascent and descent of the spinal axis, thus accomplishing a complete circuit of the universe, an inner 'cosmic year'. This practice not only interiorizes cosmic space but repeats the complex cycles of the universe in an ideal and accelerated manner within the body.

Other yogic practices assimilate the *āsanas* to living creatures; the *Gheraṇḍa Saṁhitā* affirms that there are as many yoga postures as there are animals and plants in the universe.[28] Eliade suggests that a fundamental cosmic identification of the yogi is that with a plant;[29] fixed in *āsana*, senses and mind focused on one point, the yogi becomes like an ever-verdant tree, firmly rooted alongside the stream of life, the flow of *prāṇa* in *suṣumnā* (compare the biblical image of the 'wise man': Psalm 1:3). But the basic plant symbol is that of the lotus blossom: although its roots are in the mud, its spotless petals float above the surface of the water; the yogi who is 'freed while living' remains at the highest level of consciousness while yet in the world. Although Yogananda customarily meditated in the 'lotus posture', with the right foot upon the left thigh and the left foot upon the right thigh, he invited his Western disciples to assume an erect, stable, and easier seated posture on a hard chair or bench, with the feet upon the floor and the hands resting on the thighs or folded in the lap. In fact, yoga is not postures, but meditation, and the only bodily pose required is that which simultaneously facilitates both relaxation and wakefulness.

Further cosmic-corporeal identifications include the assimilation of the various 'breaths' or *prāṇa*-currents to the winds that breathe over the surface of the earth. This identification of the life-breath with the winds is frequently found in the Upanishads and of course in the Bible.[30] In a similar way, the elements of earth, water, fire, air, and ether are identified with the centers of consciousness or *cakras*, the earth center being that at the base of the spine, followed by the water center at the urogenital level, etc.[31]

However, the yogic quest for 'cosmic consciousness' is not a mere immersion in Nature. Tantrism, while aiming at the spiritualization of human existence, maintains a certain tension in its understanding of the body-world relationship. Human destiny, according to tantric yoga, is not to escape from the world and from *saṁsāra* or profane existence, but to rise above the dualities of microcosm-macrocosm, of body and universe, of *nirvāṇa* and *saṁsāra*. The yogis of Kashmir explain the body-world relationship by identifying the evolution of human consciousness with the emanation of the universe from divine consciousness by means of God's multiform power or *śaktis*. These 'energies of God', which are the instrumental cause of the illusory separation between spirit and cosmos, are also the means for entering into a liberated manner of being in the world. United with God, who has freely manifested in the world without dividing the divine nature, a perfected yogi is freed for self-expression in the world.[32]

This self-expression of the yogi also involves the relationship with other persons. Especially in Buddhist Tantrism, but also in important Hindu texts, a sign of perfection is one's renunciation of perfection, in order to dedicate oneself to the welfare and liberation of others (the *bodhisattva* ideal).[33] The *Bhagavad-Gītā* teaches that "the greatest yogi is the one for whom others' pleasure and pain is the yogi's own pleasure and pain" (6:32). According to the *Kulārṇava Tantra*, the yogi "should do good to all beings as if they were the yogi's own self: *ātmavat sarvabhūtebhyo ḥitaṁ kuryāt.*" Abhinavagupta, the tenth-century Kashmiri master, affirms that one who is united to God is concerned only for the welfare of others.[34]

From these texts and above all from the teachings of my *guru*, Jesus, I know that the freedom I seek through yoga cannot be total indifference, an absolute 'freedom-from'; it is above all a 'freedom-for', characterized by compassion toward all beings that suffer in the bonds of *saṁsāra*. Although some tantric texts declare that the perfected yogi is bound by no law (theoretically one may kill a brahmin or have sex with the guru's spouse); yet in practice the highest moral perfection is always demanded of a yogi, not as the observance of a law but as the effortless expression of perfect freedom and compassion. Of course, there may be a symbolic or subtle sense in these examples: the 'brahmin-slayer' is one who has transcended the need for ritual sanctification, and the guru's 'spouse' is in reality the guru's *śakti*, the energy of God dwelling within the disciple's own body.[35]

The *Vijñānabhairava Tantra* describes a practice for transcending the microcosm-macrocosm duality.[36] This exercise is based on the conviction that both the individual's embodiment and the cosmic body or universe proceed from the divine consciousness by means of the evolving energies of God. The yogi strives to see this double embodiment in a vision of totality and equality by neutralizing the outgoing and incoming breaths and *prāṇa*-currents. The outer senses are disciplined, not by deadening them, but by refining their sensitivity, so that even 'the touch of an ant' can propel the yogi's consciousness to the highest state of joy. The Tantra also affirms that sexual union, understood as a yogic practice, can be an efficacious means for reaching the unitive consciousness of embodiment in the cosmos. However, the sex act by itself is only an exterior and gross image of the higher union (*maithuna*, coitus) that takes place within the yogi's own body, through the ascent of *kuṇḍalinī* to the 'abode of God', the 'thousand-petaled lotus' at the crown of the head.

Any profound human relationship, such as, for example, the joy of seeing a long-absent friend, can lead to the identification of the yogi's consciousness with the perfect joy of God. The same holds true for the pleasures of food and drink, of music and dance: if the yogi immediately focuses his mind on the essence of the gross joy, it becomes a support for the experience of the subtle joy of union with God. This yogic practice involves a continual rupture of planes between gross and subtle levels of consciousness. From the whole context of the Tantra and from subsequent tradition, it is clear that the perception of supreme joy in the moments of human wonder and delight requires a profound purification and refinement of the yogi's senses and emotions.

Maṇḍala and Tantric Iconography

The joys of music and of physical movement, like dancing or riding an elephant, can be employed in a yogic manner; in the same way, pictorial images are a potent means to the unification of consciousness. Tantric iconography usually takes the form of *maṇḍalas*, symmetrical diagrams based on concentric squares, circles, and triangles. Images of deities, animals, etc., are often inscribed within the geometrical figures. *Maṇḍalas* have an important ritual function, which remains implicit even in the purely meditative use of these icons. The complex *maṇḍala* symbolism closely unites the yogi's awareness of the body, the universe, and ritual actions.

The Sanskrit term *maṇḍala* means 'circle', and in Tibetan texts the word is translated as either 'center' or 'circumference'.[37] In fact, the basis of *maṇḍala* symbolism lies precisely in the tension between circumference and center. The graphic elements added to the icon facilitate the mental union of outer and inner space, and meditations on the *maṇḍala* usually follow the sequence of a 'march toward the center'.

The original use of *maṇḍalas* was probably in initiatory rites, and when inscribed on permanent materials (canvas, stone, etc., rather than colored sand and string), they became aids to a continued, meditative initiation.[38] In effect, the *maṇḍala* is a schematized temple, often in competition with the places of official, brahmanic worship. It constitutes as sacred any place whatever; the gods depicted in some *maṇḍalas* become truly present, just as they did in the vedic sanctuaries; for when a yogi meditates on a *maṇḍala*, it becomes the 'center of the world'.[39] Hence it is also a symbolic cosmos, a paradisiacal world depicted upon a flat surface as on a transcendent plane, patterned symmetrically with divine presences, ornamented with idealized flowers and gems, and guarded against evil influences by gates, labyrinths, and graveyards.[40]

Buddhist *maṇḍalas* are usually more elaborate, containing images of deities and *bodhisattvas* ('pre-incarnations' of the Buddha), often engaged in various symbolic actions. These divinities are not personal objects of worship in the ordinary sense; their meaning is 'psychologized' in the texts, so that they represent the states of consciousness that the yogi must experience on the way of *sādhana*.[41]

A typical Hindu *maṇḍala* is the *yantra* ('instrument'), which sums up tantric symbolism in purely geometrical form.[42] The *yantra* contains a series of variously-sized isosceles triangles inscribed within a circle around a central dot (*bindu*), forming a fourteen-pointed star. Five triangles point downward, symbolizing the *yoni* ('vagina') or feminine principle (*śakti*), and four point upward, symbolizing the male principle, the *liṅga* ('phallus') of Shiva. Gazing upon the central dot, which represents the undifferentiated unity of consciousness, I perceive each triangle separately from the others; by thus mentally unmaking the pattern, I reconstitute its primal unity in the *bindu* and experience the 'coincidence of opposites' in the meditative union of male and female principles. The *yantra* is divisible only along its vertical axis; divided horizontally, the parts are asymmetrical. This vertical orientation of the diagram, along with its male-female symbolism, makes it a pattern for the ascending movement of *kuṇḍalinī* interpreted as both coitus and sacrifice.

The *maṇḍala* described by Abhinavagupta makes this symbolic meaning even more obvious. Its central feature is the emblem of

Shiva, the trident. The shaft represents the spinal axis of the body; the various ornaments on the shaft represent the centers of consciousness or *cakras*, and the prongs, pointing upward, symbolize the union of male and female: the central prong of the trident is the *liṅga* and the two curved prongs on either side are the encompassing *yoni*.[43]

Paramahansa Yogananda's *maṇḍala* transforms Shiva's trident into a three-petaled lotus flower. At the center is a circular emblem showing a five-pointed star upon a dark blue ground, rimmed in gold. The emblem resembles the Christian-Trinitarian symbolism present in the decorative iconography of the Syrian Christians in South India. Jesus is called the 'morning star': "You will do well to pay attention to this [the voice of the Father] as to a lamp shining in a dark place, until the day dawns and the morning star rises in your hearts" (II Peter 1:19; cf. Revelation 22:16: "I, Jesus, am the bright and morning star"). The ring of golden flames is the Holy Spirit, which in Syrian hymnody is the 'feminine' in God (in the language of Jesus, the word 'Spirit', *ruḥ*, is grammatically feminine). Yogananda promised that, with the practice of Kriya Yoga, the triadic symbol would manifest spontaneously to the meditator's inner sight.

Maṇḍala symbolism unites the world, the body, and all religious actions. Viewed from above, any temple is a *maṇḍala*; when the body is viewed from a point above the head, the *cakras* coalesce to form a single *maṇḍala*, the 'thousand-petaled lotus'. In the *maṇḍala* the yogi contemplates the cosmos in its basic polarity, that is, the male-female principles and their various manifestations; by projecting the *maṇḍala* upon the body, the yogi unites flesh and cosmos in the sacrificial ascent, which is also the 'mystical marriage' in which all opposites coincide.

Time

The third factor in the tantric way of realization can be understood from the other two. Both body and cosmos are grounded in the category of space, but the concept of being-in-the-world includes the category of time as the measure of movement within space. If there is a single metaphysic implicit in Tantrism, it is certainly 'energic' rather than 'mechanistic'; Tantrism deals more with values than with substances, with process rather than static structure, with relations rather than essences. What moves in space is energy, and energy in turn arises from the separation and convergence of the pairs of opposites in the universe.

Time, for the tantric yogis, is both the condition of bondage and a means for liberation from bondage. Yoga literally 'takes time'; all its practices, whether mental or physical, involve repeated actions driving a developmental process. However, the yogis do not limit the attainment of perfect freedom to this process. Even though the progressive use of practical means is the normal way, yogis dream of an instantaneous and spontaneous liberation, consisting in the sudden 'recognition' of freedom as a given and as present from the very start.

This contrast between 'practice' and 'recognition' is basic to Abhinavagupta and his school in eleventh-century Kashmir.[44] The three 'modes' of the divine energy (the *śaktis* of will, consciousness, and action) correspond to the three basic 'ways' of yoga: the 'divine', the 'energic', and the 'particular'. In Abhinavagupta's yoga, practice is inseparable from 'grace', or the descent of *śakti* upon the yogi.[45] In virtue of the *śakti* of action, I employ the 'particular' means, such as ritual, physical discipline, and breath control. By the gift of the *śakti* of consciousness, I engage in the 'energic' practice of meditation on inner lights and sounds. Finally, moved by the will-*śakti*, I enter the 'divine' way of immediate intuition; in an indivisible moment of time, by a single and simple interior act of conformity of my will to God's, I realize true freedom in love. At least once in my life, I have experienced this intuition, and its effects abide in me to this day.

Beyond all means lies a 'fourth way', which is 'no way'; my very existence is a spontaneous, pure, and undivided act in which 'union with God' is not an end to be attained, because there is no means nor a user of means, only God. Nor do I experience the descent of *śakti*, because the energies and God are distinct no more, and they dwell at the center of my very existence. But even then, says Abhinavagupta, the ultimate reality is not static consciousness, but movement, vibration, *spanda*. The division of consciousness into *śaktis* and *tattvas* or elemental essences that proceed from the *śaktis* does not contradict the perfect unity of consciousness itself. The supreme nature is the One who both embraces unicity and multiplicity, stillness and vibration, and transcends their distinction.[46] But before reaching this mystical limit where time as bondage or as condition for liberation is no more, I must 'take time' and use time, engage continually in the practice of yogic or other means, and continue my experiment in faith.

Breath and Mantra

We measure time according to rhythms in the cosmos and within the body; the yogi strives to control these rhythms in order to control and eventually transcend the consciousness of time. The key to this control is breath. The connection between our moods (in the widest sense), our breathing, and our awareness of passing time is perfectly obvious. Yet it seems that only the yogis of India have used the breath as a basis for spiritual realization through conscious exercise. The principle of breath-control is the same as that which governs all of yoga: the coincidence of opposites. In this case, the yogi transcends the opposition between the incoming and outgoing breaths, and that between breathing and speaking.

The seers of the Upanishads saw the physical impossibility of breathing in and breathing out at the same time, or of uttering sounds and drawing breath simultaneously, as a sign of the dualities inherent in the profane condition of sentient beings.[47] Thus the unification of the breaths and the union of breath and speech is the yogic key to the realization of self as Spirit. The unification of the breaths can be achieved only by the elimination of their alternating rhythm, that is, by the suspension of breathing itself. Some popular yoga manuals propose the technique of forced retention of air, but this is not a true *kumbhaka* or suspension. The incessant rhythm of respiration is halted only when the yogi's consciousness is freed from time: when my biological clock is so altered that time no longer passes for me, only then do I abide in the indivisible moment of infinite duration between breathing out and breathing in.

As a means to the altered awareness of time, or rather, the awareness of self beyond time, you may use the mental projection of various time-intervals upon the respiratory cycle, as taught by Kashmir's great yogi Abhinavagupta.[48] Conceive of each breath, which normally has a limited duration, as moving in rhythm with progressively longer cosmic cycles: one breath takes an hour, a day, a year. Couple this mental exercise with the physical reduction of the respiratory tempo, placing its normally autonomous and often irregular function under constant control. But in addition to this mental projection, take special care to cause the breath, whatever its tempo, to flow in an uninterrupted cycle: this 'circular breathing', where the transition from in-breath to out-breath and vice verse is so even as to be almost imperceptible, makes the respiratory process so stable as to seem 'static'.

The suspension of breath is not a forced apnea but the unification of the 'inner breath' or *kuṇḍalinī*, as it moves from the base of the spine to the crown of the head, and from the periphery of the body to the heart. Link the exercise of breath control to the experience of a 'current' that flows along the body's vertical axis, so that while breathing in, the will orders the energy to rise, and while breathing out, orders it to descend. Thus you exercise control over breath and energy by focusing on different levels: on the physical breath, on the inner energies of the body, and on the consciousness of being in the body, the universe, and time.

Yogis also break free of time by breaking down the barriers between breath and speech, and between speech and thought. Some Western philosophers have emphasized the link between language and time (see Martin Heidegger); others hold that we create our world by language, when we talk about the world, explain it, and relate things and events to ourselves. Speech is an ordering factor in our experience of time; we note time, keep time with words and with numbers, which are the translation of abstract quantity into words.

The psychological connection between words and the experience of being in the world and in time is accepted implicitly by Tantrism, but the tantric yogis go one step further. Words themselves are sounds, and sounds are vibrations in a certain medium. The 'energic metaphysics' implied in the Tantras links the sounds of words with the ground of reality itself, which is vibratory energy, *spanda*. For the Kashmiri school, there is no break in the continuity between 'lower' vibratory phenomena, such as spoken words, and the highest, even the consciousness of God, which they conceive as a vibration of an infinitely high frequency.

The yogis make use of this metaphysical link between words and the divine consciousness by the practice of *mantra*. The term itself is derived from the verbal root *man-* ('think', 'perform mental actions') and the ending *-tra* ('instrument'); a *mantra* is thus a 'mental tool', an 'instrument of thought'. More specifically, it is an instrument for modifying the thought-process itself, for altering the state of consciousness. *Mantra* accomplishes this end by breaking down the ordinary connection between speech and thought, the link of conceptual meaning.

An extended phrase of the Vedas or the invocation of an object of devotion may bear some meaning for our intellect, but when broken down into its component syllables (a mnemonic exercise drilled into young brahmins) the resultant syllables are *bījas*, 'sound-seeds', and these are the true *mantras*, beyond names and concepts. Yogananda took from the *Bhāgavata Pūrāṇa* a devotional phrase in honor of Krishna: *oṁ namo bhagavate vāsudevāya*, and having broken it down into its twelve syllables, he instructed his disciples to mentally project one syllable upon each of the successive *cakras*, six ascending with the incoming breath and six descending with the outgoing breath.

The *bīja-mantras*, completely detached from all cultic or devotional texts, are the vowels, accompanied only by the aspirate (*h*), sibilant (*s*), or nasal (*ṁ*) phonemes. The greatest of these is, of course, *oṁ*, a word that in classical Sanskrit can have the meaning of 'yes', but which affirms more than just a positive answer to a question. The

Upanishads already identify this word with the very essence of the Absolute *Brahman* (see *Māṇḍūkya Upanishad*), and they associate the creaturely essence with its grammatical opposite, *na*, 'not'. Hence human language about God can only be *neti-neti*: God is not this, not that. *Oṁ* is sometimes spelled *aum*, in accordance with the scientific phonology of the ancient Sanskrit grammarians, who recognized that the original vowels were three: *a*, *i*, and *u*; *o* resulted from the fusion of *a* and *u*, and *e* was a monophthong derived from the fused diphthong *ai*.

The primal *bīja-mantra* is the 'short' *a*, the neutral vowel-sound represented in the international phonetic alphabet by the 'turned e': ə, as in the American pronunciation of 'was': *wəz*, or written like 'u' in the word 'sun'. The *Vijñānabhairava* and other Tantras teach the basic breath-*kriyā*: *haṁ-saḥ*, in which you mentally accompany the incoming breath with the syllable *haṁ*, and the outgoing with *saḥ*.[49] Note that the nasalized *aṁ* is like the sound of the French article *un*, or like the exclamation of someone suddenly roused from sleep: *Hunh*?! The syllable *saḥ* is like the word 'sun' with the 'n' replaced by a soft 'h' sound. Yogananda, who was from West Bengal, pronounced the *haṁ-saḥ mantra* with his Bengali accent: '*hong-sau*'. More important than the slight difference in pronunciation is the avoidance of an inversion of the *mantra* as *so'haṁ*, which re-introduces a conceptual meaning from the Upanishads: "I am He." However sacred this text may be, the value of a yogic *mantra* lies in its universality and its freedom from ties to ritual and philosophy.

Once again, this practice, which is an integral, albeit preliminary, practice of Kriya Yoga, entails the discipline of calm, 'circular' breathing, without any halting or glottal 'click' between in-breath and out-breath. Upon the incoming breath mentally project the syllable *haṁ*, and on the outgoing the syllable *saḥ*; do not vocally pronounce the syllables, but maintain them in the mind during the respective phase of breathing. Visualize the *kuṇḍalinī* ascending with the in-breath and descending with the out-breath.

To borrow a poetic phrase of T. S. Eliot, the *bīja-mantras* are "raids on the ineffable"; they break the bonds that tie human language to the everyday levels of consciousness. Non-cultic *mantras* correspond to certain 'mental vibrations' or psychic resonances stimulated by certain types of yogic experience. As I consciously direct *prāṇa* upward along the cerebro-genital axis, the experience is 'crystalized', as it were, by its association with a particular syllable. Thus the syllable becomes a tool for re-evoking the experience. The monosyllabic 'concentration' of the *bīja-mantra* raises its vibratory 'frequency' in harmony with the elevation of consciousness and makes it an instrument for transcending time. It raises thought beyond the ordinary, everyday language by which we note and express time, and it dissociates our consciousness from the rhythms or vibrations that are the measure of time. The *mantra* becomes the key to entry into those higher states of consciousness in which existence in the body, the world, and time becomes the context of perfect freedom.

---

1 Cf. Mircea Eliade, *Yoga, Immortality and Freedom* (Princeton N.J.: Princeton U. Press, 1969), p. 204; cf. also Eliade, "Le probème des origines du Yoga," in Jacques Masui, ed., *Yoga, science de l'homme intégral* (Paris: Editions Cahiers du Sud, 1953), pp. 11-20. Cf. Jan Gonda, *Die Religionen Indiens*, Vol. 2, Der juengere Hinduismus, Die Religionen der Menschheit 12 (Stuttgart: W. Kohlhammer, 1964), pp. 26-52; Maurice Maupilier, *Le Yoga et l'homme d'occident* (Paris: Editions du Seuil, 1974), pp. 154-168; John Woodroffe, *Śakti and Śākta: Essays and Addresses* (1927; reprint Madras: Ganesh, 1969) *passim*.

2 Today's historians of Indian proto-history are reluctant to speak of an 'invasion'; what probably took place were successive waves of migrations, which met, now with more, now with less resistance; cf.

Rajesh Kochar, *The Vedic People: Their History and Geography* (Hyderabad: Orient Longman, 2000).

3 Cf. Eliade, *Yoga*, p. 201; and "Le problème des origines du yoga," Masui, pp. 11-20.

4 Walter A. Fairservis, *The Roots of Ancient India: The Archeology of Early Indian Civilization* (New York: Macmillan, 1971), pp. 258-259.

5 This would be either the *baddhakonāsana* or the *mulabandhāsana*; cf. B. K. S. Iyengar, *Light on Yoga: Yoga Dīpikā* (New York: Schocken, 1966), pp. 197-198.

6 Fairservis, pp. 176-277; cf. Eliade, *Yoga*, p. 355.

7 Cf. Eliade, "Le problème," Masui, p. 19.

8 Cf. Eliade, *Yoga*, pp. 202-203.

9 Cf. idem, pp. 203-204; cf. John Woodroffe, *Introduction to Tantra Sastra*, 6th ed. (Madras: Ganesh, 1973), pp. 41-42. According to the *Mahānirvāṇa Tantra*, the Vedas are fruitless like a barren woman, and their *mantras* are useless; only the tantric *mantras* are efficacious; cf. John Woodroffe, *Tantra of the Great Liberation (Mahānirvāṇa Tantra)* (1913; reprint New York: Dover, 1972) pp. 16-17. For other arguments, see Lama Anagarika Govinda, *Foundations of Tibetan Mysticism* (1960; reprint New York: Weiser, 1974); see also the Buddhist tantric apologetics cited by Shashi Bhushan Dasgupta, *An Introduction to Tantric Buddhism* (1937; reprint Berkeley, Calif.: Shambhala, 1974), pp. 179-198.

10 Cf. Kees W. Bolle, *The Persistence of Religion: An Essay on Tantrism and Sri Aurobindo's Philosophy* (Leiden: Brill, 1971), p. 65.

11 Cf. Eliade, *Yoga*, pp. 249-254; cf. Agehananda Bharati, *The Tantric Tradition* (London: Rider, 1965), pp. 164-180.

12 Cf. Bharati, pp. 16-21.

13 Cf. Eliade, *Yoga*, p. 293.

14 Cf. Jnanavatar Swami Sri Yukteswar Giri, *Kaivalya Darśanam: The Holy Science* (1894; reprint Los Angeles: Self-Realization Fellowship, 1972); cf. Paramahansa Yogananda, *Autobiography of a Yogi*, With a preface by W. Y. Evans-Wentz...

(New York: Philosophical Library, 1946; revised reprint Los Angeles: Self-Realization Fellowship, 1972); quotations will be made from the original edition, available on several Internet sites, but the page numbers will refer to the 1972 edition.

15 E.g. *Chāndogya Upanishad* 3:16-17; 5:18-24; *Kauṣitaki Upanishad* 2:5; *Bhagavad-Gītā* 4:24-33; cf. Eliade, *Yoga*, pp. 111-114; Franklin Edgerton, *The Beginnings of Indian Philosophy* (Cambridge, MA: Harvard U. Press, 1965), pp. 67-68.

16 Cf. Eliade, *Yoga*, p. 200; Bolle, p. 41.

17 Herbert V. Guenther, *The life and Teachings of Naropa* (1963; reprint London: Oxford U. Press, 1974), Introduction, p. 1.

18 Cf. Kanti Chandra Pandey, *Abhinavagupta: An Historical and Philosophical Study* (Varanasi: Chowkhamba Sanskrit Series, 1963), pp. 149-150; see below, Appendix I, for a complete list of the primary tantric sources cited in this book; wherever possible, I have translated the text of my quotations from the original Sanskrit.

19 Eliade, *Yoga*, p. 204.

20 Cf. idem, pp. 95-96 and 362.

21 Cf. *Śiva Sūtras* 3:26-28 (Pereira, p. 363) and the teachings of the Tibetan master Gambopa (in Guenther, *The Jewel Ornament*, p. 18).

22 Cf. *Gheraṇḍa Saṃhitā*, in Theos Bernard, *Haṭha Yoga: The Report of a Personal Experience* (1950; reprint London:Rider, 1968), p. 18, note 7.

23 Cf. Govinda, pp. 137-139, 143, and 175.

24 See, for example, the *Ṣaṭcakranirūpaṇa*: text and translation in John Woodroffe, *The Serpent Power* (1918; reprint Madras: Ganesh, 1973), pp. 317-479.

25 Cf. Agehananda Bharati, pp. 112-113 and 246.

26 Cf. Carl Sagan, *The Cosmic Connection: An Extraterrestrial Perspective* (New York, Dell: 1973).

27 Cf. Eliade, *Yoga*, pp. 97-98, 240, and 244.

28 Cf. Bernard, p. 22.

29 Cf. Eliade, *Yoga*, pp. 54 and 66-67; cf. also *Ṣaṭcakranirūpaṇa*, in Woodroffe, *The Serpent Power*, p. 317.

30 E.g. *Bṛhadāraṇyaka Upanishad* 3:7:2; *Chāndogya Up*. 3:13:1-5; Ezekiel 37, etc.

31 Cf. *Yogatattva Upanishad* 84-104; trans. Jean Varenne, *Les Upanishads du Yoga* (Paris: Gallimard, 1971), pp. 62-85.

32 Cf. Raniero Gnoli, *Luce delle sacre scritture (Tantrāloka) di Abhinavagupta* (Turin: UTET, 1972), pp. 33-37.

33 See the abundant expressions of this ideal in Buddhist literature, as in the life of Milarepa, who successively converted to nonviolence a hunter, his dog, and the deer: in Garma C. C. Chang, trans., *The Hundred Thousand Songs of Milarepa* (1962; reprint New York: Harper Colophon, 1970), pp. 142-153.

34 Cf. *Tantrāloka* 2:39, in Gnoli, *Luce delle sacre scritture*, p. 117.

35 Cf. Abhinavagupta, *Paramārthasāra* 70 (p. 86).

36 In Lilian Silburn, *Le Vijñāna Bhairava*, pp. 107-117.

37 Cf. Eliade, *Yoga*, p. 219; see also Giuseppe Tucci, *The Theory and Practice of the Mandala* (1961; reprint New York: Weiser, 1969); P. H. Pott, *Yoga and Yantra* (The Hague: Nijhoff, 1966).

38 Cf. Eliade, *Yoga*, pp. 221-227.

39 Cf. Tucci, p. 51; Eliade, *Yoga*, pp. 220 and 225.

40 Cf. Eliade, *Yoga*, pp. 222-223.

41 Cf. Govinda, pp. 110-111; W. Y. Evans-Wentz, *Tibet's Great Yogi Milarepa: A Biography From the Tibetan* (1951; reprint London: Oxford U. Press, 1972), p. 141 and note 2 ibid.

42 Cf. Tucci, pp. 47-48; Pott, pp. 28-50.

43 Cf. Raniero Gnoli, trans., *Abhinavagupta: Essenza dei Tantra (Tantrasāra)* (Turin: Boringhieri, 1960), pp. 331-334.

44 Cf. *Paramārthasāra*, pp. 41-47; *Mahārthamañjarī*, pp. 21-23 and 44-45.

45 Cf. *Vijñāna Bhairava*, p. 25.

46 Cf. Abhinavagupta, *Tantrāloka* chapters 2-5, pp. 113-207.

47 For example, *Kauṣītaki-Brāhmaṇa Upanishad* 2:5.

48 Abhinavagupta drew his technique of projecting successively longer time-cycles onto breathing from the *Kālacakra Tantra*; cf. Gnoli, *Luce delle sacre scritture*, pp. 208-237; *Essenza dei Tantra*, pp. 136-151; Eliade, *Yoga*, p. 271.

49 Cf. *Vijñānabhairava Tantra* 155-156; Silburn, p. 170.

Chapter III

The Experience of Symeon the New Theologian

In the last chapter, we looked at some of the constants in the history of tantric yoga, the elements of the *sādhana* or quest for perfection common to the various schools of Tantrism. *Mantra*, *maṇḍala*, the interior sacrifice, the cosmic consciousness that unites individual embodiment with the great body of the universe, are used by yogis who aim at ends that they express in different ways. Yogis often talk about their experience using similar terms grounded in basic, archetypal symbols, but they understand their experience in the light of their 'faith', that is, the idea and ideal of the ultimate end as proposed by scriptures, the guru, and their general religious culture. This vision of the end is the meaning that every yogi reads into the practice and experience of yoga.

Something similar happened to a great Christian mystic, Symeon, called 'the New Theologian': as a young seeker he began to have a series of experiences, which, as he described them, seem analogous to the 'awakening of *kuṇḍalinī*', but Symeon read into his experiences the meaning given him by his Christian faith.

The light in which he was bathed and the fire in which he was immersed were, he said, "God, or the glory of God." They were nothing less than an uncreated grace, God acting directly and immediately on his body and in his soul. Symeon narrated these events and laid out the meaning he found in them; a later theologian, Gregory Palamas, developed the testimony of Symeon and other hesychasts into a theology of the 'divine energies', communicated eternally within the life of the Trinity ('Father, Son, Spirit') and shared in time with human beings, thus making us sharers in the divine nature (cf. II Peter 1:4).[1]

Symeon experienced God's uncreated energies and spoke of them in symbolic terms that seem to echo those of the Tantras. If we share Symeon's faith, we can understand his experience as he did, but we cannot identify, much less judge, the meaning that the yogis found in their experience. They may have seen the same light and fire within them, but beyond this analogy we cannot go; we profoundly respect each one's experience and humbly accept our unknowing with regard to its ultimate meaning, which only the experiencer can know.

Symeon was born in the mid-tenth century CE in Paphlagonia (an Asian region of modern Turkey, along the southern coast of the Black Sea). At age twenty-seven, he entered the great monastery of Stoudios in Constantinople (modern Istanbul). The community did not accept him, but an elder monk, who was his 'spiritual father', also named Symeon, took him to a small monastery on the outskirts of the city. There, in the space of three years, Symeon was clothed with the monastic robes and ordained a priest. The monks elected him as their abbot, but the zealous, young superior had to deal with a community content with the external formalities of monastic life without much commitment to its spiritual goal.

There followed a slow war of attrition between abbot and monks. Symeon also made enemies in the imperial and patriarchal courts; the rebellious monks played on this animosity, and under the accusation of doctrinal and disciplinary errors, Symeon was forced to resign his office and leave the city. Although the civil and ecclesiastical authorities finally rehabilitated him, Symeon refused to return to Constantinople, and after a few more years of writing and contemplation in his hermitage, he died in 1022.[2]

In this and the following chapters, I place Symeon's experience alongside that of the tantric yogis, but I will not be analyzing his theology nor comparing it to Hindu or Buddhist doctrines. I will take what he said about his experience and examine its psychological structure and symbolic expression, in order to find out what he understood to be its underlying meaning. This meaning flowed from his faith in the Bible and the tradition of the Orthodox Church.[3] At the same time, his mystical experience transcended concepts and penetrated through and beyond the dogmatic formulas of Christianity into the mystery these formulas conceptualize. Symeon experienced a God beyond all names and all essences, even as he struggled to retranslate his experience back into the language of his faith tradition.

A Mystic with a Mission

For Symeon, all Christians are, or should be, mystics; that is, their faith ought to give them a new vision, a different consciousness of themselves, other persons, the universe, and God. If we learn to see all things in a different light, our faith in God's self-revelation will penetrate to the deepest levels, transforming not only our external behavior, but also our motives, thought patterns, and emotional reflexes. While transformation of consciousness by faith is the essence of Christian mysticism, it is also true that our transformation does not always emerge on the level of verbal or waking consciousness; in other words, we cannot always explain, even to ourselves, what faith does to us. Those who are commonly called 'mystics' are individuals who are able to translate their inner transformation into words and symbols that others can understand.

Symeon the New Theologian was without question an exceptional person; perhaps no one else in the history of Christianity has come closer to expressing the inexpressible. There is also something a bit frightening in what he reveals to us about his experience of God; glorious it is, but uncanny and apparently distant from ordinary life. This fact, coupled with the cultural remoteness of a man who lived in a vanished empire a thousand years ago, does not make him immediately attractive.

It is often easier for us to relate to Hindu and Buddhist sages, of our own time or of ages past, than to Christian mystics; we are sometimes more willing to listen to the former than to the latter. If Symeon does not always speak our language, if we hear a harsh tone in his writings, and if he is occasionally over-insistent on the obligation to become mystics, we should try to remember the sense of urgency with which he wrote, and his genuine sincerity in fulfilling what he believed to be his mission: to awaken every Christian to the possibility of seeing the light of Christ in this life.

It is true that there is not an equal proportion between the subjective and objective elements in Symeon's faith and theology. Yet he always strove to maintain these elements in balance, and perhaps he succeeded about as well as any other mystic in the history of Christianity. In any case, we can be grateful to Symeon for his 'subjectivity', the autobiographical aspect of his writings that makes it possible for us to understand and share his experience.

The First Vision

Symeon's life and thought were given their essential form by his 'mystical initiation', the sudden and overwhelming crisis that befell him at the age of twenty.

He was employed in the imperial court, charged with the personal affairs of one of the patricians, a relative of his. Spiritually restless, he went looking for a guide, whom he found in the person of an old monk, Symeon Eulabes, who would later be the master of the novice Symeon at the monastery of Stoudios. The monk gave him some books to read and counseled him never to silence the voice of his conscience.

Symeon's life seemed to be moving in two different directions: toward a secular career at the imperial court and toward life in a monastery. For a while, he tried to respond to both attractions at once, living by day like the other young men at court, while devoting a good portion of his nights to prayer.

Perhaps misunderstanding his spiritual father's counsel never to say no to his conscience, Symeon spent hours at prayer every evening; he forced himself to remain immobile, erect or prostrate on the floor, giving vent to intense religious emotions and reciting endless prayers to Christ the Savior and the Mother of God. At midnight he retired to sleep. The next day he continued to live his usual, worldly life.[4]

Symeon had no problem with this divided existence. His night vigils seemed easy, and to increase their length cost him little effort. But one evening something happened for which he was totally unprepared. Nothing in his religious formation had led him to expect the kind of phenomena that overwhelmed him.[5]

Suddenly there was light. The night became bright as day, and the light filled the room.

"It seemed to me as if I had left the body, the house, and the entire world behind," he wrote; "I lost all awareness of my surroundings and forgot whether I was at home or even indoors."

In other words, Symeon was in ecstasy, and yet he was careful to avoid saying he was literally outside the body, preferring Paul's expression: "whether he was in the body or out of it, I know not; God knows" (II Corinthians 12:2-3). The vision that ended the ecstasy was for him the most important part of the experience.

"There, as if in heaven, at the very summit of your Godhead, I beheld in awe (for so you judged me worthy) my saintly teacher, standing in the presence of your glory. He was not crowned or brilliantly robed, nor was his appearance altered. I saw him there, in heaven, just like he was when I saw him every day."[6]

This final and culminating moment of the vision revealed two things: first, that his salvation depended on the help and guidance he was receiving from the elder Symeon; and second, that the transforming effects of the light do not cancel the outward, familiar aspect of the mystic's humanity. In other words, the light of God elevates the human and the everyday and makes them share in the divine nature.

The Second Vision

The first ecstatic experience had no lasting effect on his life; on the contrary, he confesses, "I came to despise what I had gotten so cheaply, even forgetting the vision itself."[7]

Symeon continued to visit his teacher, and slowly his monastic vocation took root and began to grow in the secret of his soul. After six years he finally entered the monastery, where he was placed under the direction of the elder Symeon. The novice threw himself into intense asceticism and spiritual training, moved by desire for the high mystical states that the old monk described to him. Faith, not self-conscious spiritual vanity, motivated him now.[8]

One day the novice accompanied his teacher on a trip into town; they returned tired and hungry. The old monk began to eat, but the novice was troubled, saying to himself, "If I eat at this hour, I won't feel like praying tonight."

The wise elder told him to go ahead and eat, reminding him, "If God had not wanted to have mercy on you, he would not have sent you to me."

Later, Symeon went to his room and began to pray as usual. Once again the light appeared, suddenly and unexpectedly as before. Symeon was in ecstasy; his fatigue disappeared: "The light so invigorated and strengthened my weary limbs and muscles, that it seemed to me as though I were stripping off the garment of mortal flesh."

The liberation of the body was accompanied by an inner liberation: "Into my soul and senses was poured a sweetness surpassing every material taste, together with freedom and forgetfulness of all thoughts pertaining to earthly life."

He then experienced a series of inner sensations, one following distinctly from the other: "I felt a supernatural warmth, then I perceived a faint, radiant luminosity, then a breath of God entered me with my teacher's words, then a fire came forth from him and filled my heart, causing tears to spring forth in endless flow, and a fine ray flashed through my spirit faster than lightning. What appeared to me next was like a torch in the night or a small, flaming cloud, which rested on my head, as I lay face down in prayer. Then the cloud flew off, and shortly after I saw it in the heavens."[9]

In contrast with the diffuse luminosity of Symeon's first vision, the light now begins to assume more definite outlines. Symeon likens his novice years to the condition of a blind man trying to wash the scales from his eyes; he gropes about the metaphorical pool of Bethesda, splashing mud into his eyes instead of the clear water that would heal them. At a certain point, the blind man becomes aware of someone else who is washing him, accomplishing for him what he could not by his own efforts.

"You were present to me, and you seemed to be washing me in the waters, pouring them over me and immersing me into them. I beheld with wonder as lightning flashed about me and the rays of your face were mixed with the water. I was in a daze, seeing myself sprinkled with luminous water."

Symeon asked himself, "Who was doing this? Where was he? Whence had he come? I did not know; I only rejoiced as I was being bathed, growing in faith, flying on wings of hope, and ascending into heaven."[10]

Aside from the general light symbolism, the image of lightning again suggests the astonishing nature of the experience and links this passage with the other accounts of the second vision. The light has a clearer form than before and is identified with a mysterious Other, although Symeon cannot say who he is. Another symbol is that of the ascent, although sometimes it is the cloud that rises from Symeon's head to the heavens, while at other times Symeon himself ascends, "flying on wings of hope."

The Evolution of the Mystical Grace

One fact stands out in Symeon's accounts of his earlier visions: they did not bring with them an immediate understanding of their meaning. Who or what the light was did not emerge at the level of conceptual understanding. His stupor and wonder were not simply a reaction to the unfamiliarity of the visions: Symeon is making a theological statement when he says he was unable to recognize the Lord in the light. If the mystic is to recognize and understand God in his experience, God must take the initiative and tell him.

When the light first came upon Symeon, it was an unexpected wonder that filled him with amazement but with little understanding. "I did not yet realize that it was you," he wrote. "You had not yet spoken to me the secret words, 'It is I.' And so I saw you, my God, but without knowing and without believing that God is seen by a human creature, to the extent that God can be seen at all. I did not understand that the light, which appeared to me now in one way and now in another, was God or the glory of God."[11] His life thereafter became a progressive initiation into the meaning of his visions.

Symeon sought the answer in prayer: "O Lord, who could it be? Is it you?"

And the answer came: "I am the God who, for your sake, became human, and since you have sought me with all your mind, from now on you will be my brother, my fellow heir, my friend."[12]

Again Symeon takes up the metaphor of the blind man to explain his gradual initiation into the mystical light. "When you let yourself be seen by me, I became like a blind man who begins to recover his sight little by little: he first notes human shapes and then bit by bit ascertains what they are."

He explains that it is not the form itself whose shape is altered, but it is the blind man's sense of sight that is being restored. Thus he begins to see the human form as it is: all the characteristics are imprinted on his visual faculty, through which the form penetrates into the mental faculties of understanding and memory, inscribing its shape upon them.

Symeon concludes: "In a like manner, by the clear light of the Holy Spirit, you restored my sight to its integral purity. Thus by means of a progressively clearer and purer spiritual vision you appeared to me, seeming to emerge and grow brighter, and enabling me to see the shape of a form without form."[13]

Symeon does not make theological distinctions between 'natural' and 'supernatural' ends, or between 'acquired' and 'infused' contemplation. He always speaks in concrete terms of human destiny according to the intention of God revealed in Christ. It is natural for me to see the light of God's glory, but in my fallen state I need to be healed of my blindness and trained to understand what I see. This healing process is a restoration and reintegration of my original condition; at the same time, it is a realization or 'recognition' of the light of God's energies in me.

Symeon emphasizes what theology calls 'objective salvation', God's work has been fulfilled in Christ, and I need only open my spiritual eye to realize it. But just as children whose sight is normal do not recognize what they see until they are taught to distinguish the forms of things (they see large animals, for instance, but do not distinguish between horses and cows until they are taught the difference), likewise I do not immediately grasp the meaning of the light as it first appears. As I grow, I am taught by God to see, in the light, the 'form without form'; the word of God, received in faith by hearing, shapes my vision.

Elsewhere Symeon traces the development of the contemplation of light in and through his own mind and body. "When one has spent some time in the quest for this vision, without ever turning back, it all becomes clear and open; how, I do not know, nor would I know how to tell whether what is 'opened' to me is heaven, or the eye of my heart, or the one more than the other. The light itself does this, the same light that is within the house of the soul, I mean, this earthly tent; that marvelous light enters, bright beyond measure, making me light, to the extent of my natural capacity."[14]

The key word is 'open'; the symbolism of light suggests disclosure; a reality once hidden has now come to light. I cannot determine whether the 'opening' is in God or myself, nor can I, just by introspection, distinguish God's activity in me from my soul's own activity.[15] This is a case in point of 'synergy' or the dialectic of grace and human effort in the spiritual quest. There is no division of labor between God and the soul, rather a mysterious interpenetration and cooperation of two freedoms, human and divine.[16] God is the doer, of course: "The light itself does this," says Symeon, and yet grace enters into "this earthly tent," the human body, and transforms it into light.

Symeon continues: "After some time in this stage, I began little by little to regard the light, great as it was, as something familiar, as if it had already been there from the beginning. Having experienced one marvel, mystery, and vision after another, illuminated every hour by the light, I see, I know, I am initiated, I am taught."[17]

This further stage of contemplation is a permanent mystical state, a condition in which the experience of God as light is no longer a transient irruption into the everyday, involving an altered state of consciousness, but a radical transformation of the vision of reality as a whole. The human mind, bathed in light, is taught by God, but God's teaching transcends words and concepts. The meaning discovered in the light becomes the horizon of all meanings, in oneself, in others, and in the universe.

This is the ultimate penetration of the 'supernatural' into the 'natural' in this life. Symeon says: "I am in the light or united to the light, but not in a continual state of ecstasy. I see myself, my surroundings, and others as they are." Great as it is, this state is penultimate with respect to the definitive resurrection and liberation of the body. Symeon quotes Paul's great affirmation: "No eye has seen, nor ear heard, nor human heart conceived, what God has prepared for those who love him" (I Corinthians 2:9, cf. Isaiah 64:4). Symeon foresees and predicts this ultimate vision, because here and now the light dwells in him and makes him light.[18]

Symeon's summary of his mystical doctrine concludes with two capital points: first, that the highest mystical state passes beyond the condition of ecstasy into a completely transformed world where persons and things are perceived as they really are in God; second, that all mystical graces, including the highest, are ordered to a fulfillment beyond this life. Despite his emphasis on the necessity of mystical experience for all Christians, Symeon acknowledged that what we experience in this life is incomparably less than eternal glory, although the difference between the two visions is one of degree, not of kind.[19] The mystics realize this truth, precisely because they possess a foretaste of eternal glory here and now.

Symeon's Experience and the Theology of Grace

Symeon affirms that the transforming light penetrates deep into both his consciousness and his body. Awakening to the light, he recognizes a reality already present in him; progress in the vision is a growing familiarity with the light. His habitual state is not ecstatic but a transformed vision of self and world in God. He already lives the resurrection; his eye is now 'single', so that his "whole body will be full of light" (Matthew 6:22). He sees the divine light as it really is, because he has become like it (cf. I John 3:2); when he is in the light, he is the light!

While saying this, Symeon never forgets that the light is a gift, a grace, the descent of God's energy into flesh, into sinful, broken creatures, healing our blindness and illumining our darkness.

The teachers of the Eastern Church, no less than Western theologians, recognized God's freedom and initiative in the work of our liberation and illumination. "God is the doer," a disciple of Yogananda once reminded me, and then I found the same teaching in both the *Bhagavad-Gītā* and the Gospel according to John. But we are also free and responsible agents in this doing.

Having declared the essential distinction and the inseparable union of the two energies and the two wills, human and divine, in Jesus Christ, the Eastern Church had no need to develop a separate doctrine of grace. Our total nature was assumed into God, once for all, when (in its classical formulation) "the second Hypostasis of the Blessed Trinity became human (*ánthrōpos*) in the womb of the Virgin Mary"; thus nature itself became grace. The bodily resurrection of Jesus *ipso facto* resurrects human flesh, although we still await our personal resurrection. We who share the humanity of the Word-made-flesh have only to recognize, assume, and integrate the grace that our nature, in Jesus, has become. Hence we hear the great affirmation of mystical Christianity handed down from Saint Irenaeus in the second century CE to Thomas Aquinas in the thirteenth (although it is seldom repeated by today's theologians): "God became human, so that every human being might become God."

More important than the distinction between nature and grace is that between *praxis* and *theōría*. *Praxis* is the 'active life', not in the sense of corporal and spiritual works of mercy, although these are included, but as a 'struggle for virtue'. It includes all that we actively do, under the influence of grace, to reintegrate our being as spirit, soul, and body in the quest for God. Monastics emphasize ascetical practices: fasting, silence, living alone, praying at night, etc. *Praxis* also includes loving service to our neighbor, as well as what the Jesuit mystic Teilhard de Chardin called 'sanctification of passivities'.[20]

Theōría, usually translated 'contemplation', means 'vision of light'. In Christian experience it is a gift, a light from beyond, although we are not passive recipients of it; we engage our own energies in the mystical vision. For Symeon, *theōría* will not be given unless it is sought.

Symeon's lineage distinguished two kinds of contemplation: *theōría physikē*, the vision of God in created beings, and *theōría theologikē*, the vision of the Holy Trinity without any 'support' for contemplation.[21] In Symeon's visions, he experiences *theōría* as both 'gift' (the light falls unexpectedly upon him) and 'natural' (the divine image and likeness, in which God created him, shines forth). He understands God's doing in creation, redemption, and sanctification as one *oikonomia* or 'dispensation'. Since God, from eternity, wills that we see the light of the Son through the gift of the Holy Spirit, and orders our existence in time to this end, we have only to cooperate freely and actively to attain it.

Symeon's emphasis on our freedom and activity, which is that of the monastic tradition in general, does not imply any ability on our part to produce the light. The divine Bridegroom calls each soul as bride, chosen yet free, and offers her a sign of spiritual betrothal, like an engagement ring. Symeon uses this metaphor to describe his experience.

"The ring, for one who possesses it, is something ineffable, understood without being understood, grasped without being grasped, seen without being seen. It is a living, communicating, acting presence; it even acts on the one to whom it belongs. It can vanish suddenly, even though I keep it in a sealed coffer, and then, just as unexpectedly, I find it once again inside. When it is there, or when it is not, I cannot regard either its presence or absence as permanent. For when I have it, it is as if I did not, and when I do not, it is as if I did."[22]

The infused nature of contemplation does not mean only a subjective sense of passivity. On the contrary, the familiarity of the light at the highest stage of *theōría* makes the light a personal possession, an inner reality that permeates all levels of my activity and passivity. At the same time, the light is not subject to my whims; it acts upon me, and whenever I try to grasp it, the light seems to vanish, teaching me that it is always God's free gift.

God is ungraspable not only because our minds are limited but because God's existence and life are of an order totally different from existing things. A fifth-century mystic of the Eastern Church, who went by the pseudonym of 'Dionysius the Areopagite', said: "If God is, we are not; if we are, God is not," and after him, John of Damascus affirmed that God is not only above all names, but above all essences. This is called 'apophatic theology' and is typical of Eastern Church writers: we can say, not what God is, but only what God is not.[23] But there is a bridge between God's unknowability and our minds: it is God's loving condescension, not just a momentary 'descent' (*avatāra*) into creaturely form but a total assumption of human flesh and the human heart into God.

---

1 Cf. Jaroslav Pelikan, *The Spirit of Eastern Christendom*, The Christian Tradition: A History of the Development of Doctrine vol. 2 (Chicago: U. of Chicago Press, 1974), pp. 252-270.

2 After Symeon's death, his disciple Nikētas Stéthatos wrote a biography of him; see the translation by Irénée Hausherr, *Un grand mystique byzantin: Vie de Syméon le Nouveau Théologien par Nicétas Stéthatos* (Rome: Orientalia Christiana 9,45 [1928]); we will cite this work as *Vie*. See Appendix II for the list of critical editions of Symeon's writings as published in *Sources Chrétiennes* (Paris:Ed. du Cerf, 1955 ff). Here we give the abbreviations of the works: CT ("Catechetical Sermons"), EU ("Eucharists" or "Thanksgivings"), TGP ("Theological, Gnostical, and Practical Chapters"), TT ("Theological Treatises"), TE ("Treatises on Ethics"), H ("Hymns").

3 Cf. Vladimir Lossky, *The Mystical Theology of the Eastern Church* (1957; reprint London: Clarke, 1968).

4 CT 22, 75-87.

5 Stéthatos narrates the event in *Vie*, pp. 8-10.

6 Symeon tells of his initial experience three times, with slight variations: CT 6,121-131; CT 22,22-116; EU 1,100-113. He often speaks of himself in the third person, using the cover name 'George';

in my translation of the texts, I have recast the discourse in the first person.

7 Cf. CT 22,275-288; EU 1,114-116.

8 The following episodes are narrated in CT 16,7-107.

9 EU 1,131-139; Stéthatos also mentions the cloud, but in connection with the first vision: *Vie*, p. 8.

10 EU 2,148-155.

11 EU 1, 156-168.

12 EU 2,224-233.

13 EU 2,208-221.

14 TE I,12,416-424.

15 Cf. H 11,36 and 46; in H 35,4-7, Symeon prays that God may open heaven to him, or rather open his mind.

16 See Symeon's doctrine on synergy in CT 6.

17 TE I,12,424-433.

18 TE I,12,433-442; cf. TE 3.

19 Cf. EU 2, 249-254; CT 16, 138-144.

20 See Pierre Teilhard de Chardin, *Le milieu divin* (1957; reprint London: Collins, 1971), pp. 74-94.

21 Cf. Vladimir Lossky, *The Vision of God* (1963; reprint London: Faith Press, 1973), p. 47.

22 TGP 3,53.

23 Cf. Lossky, *Mystical Theology*, pp. 23-43.

Chapter IV

Symeon and the Yogis: A Vocabulary of Symbols

The language of the mystics is a raid on the ineffable, an attempt to communicate the incommunicable experience of their transformation in God. Symeon tries to express what he saw by means of symbols drawn from the Bible and grounded in our external senses.

"The saints no longer belong to themselves but to the Spirit within them, who moves them and is moved by them," he says, and then he gives a series of terms that the Bible uses to describe the Spirit's field of action: a 'pearl', a 'grain of mustard seed', 'leaven', 'water', 'fire', 'bread', a 'drink of life', a 'living spring'. He continues: "The divine life is a lamp, a nuptial bed, a bridal chamber; it is the embrace of a spouse, a friend, a sibling, a parent." And then he gives up, unable to find words to translate "what eye has not seen, nor ear heard, nor human mind conceived."[1]

Human language is based on sense experience, and our mind unites the various data into a composite impression of the world. But the 'spiritual sense' or 'new eye' is one and indivisible.[2] For this reason, the many words and symbols by which Symeon conveys his experience are closely linked among themselves. He seldom speaks of 'light' without reference to 'fire'; 'fire' is likewise associated with 'water', and the latter, as something to drink, with 'wine'. The symbol of 'wine' sums up those of 'light' and 'fire' and also suggests the 'wedding banquet', hence the erotic imagery so common in mystical literature. The 'banquet' and the 'mystical marriage' are celebrated in the 'city of God', the 'inner kingdom', which is the human heart, where created spirits unite with the uncreated Spirit.

Symeon and the tantric yogis share the conviction that the senses indeed share in the divine vision, but only insofar as they are detached from their multiple objects and focused upon that spiritual faculty whose one object, the divine energy, transcends the powers of each and all of the physical senses.[3] But the participation of our bodily senses in the activity of the one spiritual sense makes it possible and necessary to speak of the experience as a seeing, feeling, tasting, etc. This is why our consciousness of union with God is indistinguishably light, fire, wine, and embrace. As this consciousness expands outward from our heart and overflows into our embodied being, it finds expression in the various terms that Symeon and the yogis use.

'Light' Symbolism in Tantric Texts

Symeon makes it clear that 'light' is more than just a metaphor for him; it is a real fact of experience.[4] In tantric literature also, we find the same symbols used in a very concrete way, and we can suppose that they refer to actual yogic experience. Abhinavagupta (Kashmir, mid tenth to early eleventh century) is probably the greatest witness to the yogis' vision of the inner light. For Abhinavagupta, the 'clouds of doubt' are dissolved by three means: the words of the guru, mental purification through meditation, and faith in the scriptures. When these clouds vanish, he says, the yogi experiences "the rays of the Lord, whose splendor shines in the sky of the heart and, like a rising sun, destroys the darkness."[5]

The yogi neutralizes 'night and day' (the descending and ascending currents of *prāṇa*), beholds the 'great light', and enters into the 'citadel' of the heart; in this state, soul and body shine with the splendor of all the energies of God.[6] The *Mahānirvāṇa Tantra* also describes the perfected yogi as one like a 'second sun', clothed with the splendor of *brahman* (the Absolute).[7]

Abhinavagupta teaches that the yogi, by means of the 'unitive breath' (*samāna*) attains blessedness and reposes in the infinite light of all knowable things.[8] Then the 'free light' of conscious union with God is seen in the heart as a flower of many petals, in which all things converge.[9] Freedom is attained when 'the sun and the moon' unite (i.e., when the opposite currents of life-energy, *prāṇa*, enter into the central channel of the energic body, the *suṣumnā*) and dissolve into the divine consciousness, and when the 'living sun' has reached the zenith of the inner zodiac. At this point, the yogi is free and able to make others free; there is no further need of external yoga practices.[10]

Buddhist yogis also speak of their experiences in terms of light. The concept of the 'radiant mind' is already present in the Pali Canon (early sacred texts of Buddhism, dating from the fifth century BCE to the beginning of the Common Era). In Naropa and the Kagyupa school, light becomes the chief symbol of the highest spiritual state, Buddhahood or *dharmakāya* ('body of truth'), in which the body is transfigured and the mind becomes light, bliss, and paradoxical nothingness.[11] The highest perfection is always expressed as a paradox: the 'nothing' or 'voidness' (*śūnyatā*) is at the same time a fullness described as bliss (*ānanda*), as compassion (*karuṇā*), and as luminous awareness.

The ordinary human condition is like that of a lamp in a pitcher; when the teaching of a guru breaks the pitcher, the light shines forth.[12] For Milarepa's disciple Gambopa, the perfect consciousness that is Buddhahood is experienced as light. A yogi, who, at the moment of death, fixes the eye of the heart on the 'clear light', immediately attains liberation.[13] In the teachings of both Abhinavagupta and the Kagyupa school, highest consciousness, the awareness of the 'void' as light, is attained by means of the union of 'sun and moon'. Drawing the life-energy or 'vital fluid' up through the median channel, the yogi perceives various signs of progress, described in almost identical terms in a number of texts.[14]

As we learn to move the *prāṇa* through the various centers of consciousness in the body (the *cakras*, in which *prāṇa* is related to the five elements: earth, water, fire, air, ether), we experience light-phenomena characterized by vagueness and obscurity. But when the *prāṇa* is established in the median channel and reposes in the heart, the phenomena are brighter and clearer, culminating in the fusion of the two currents, ascending and descending ('sun and moon'). This succession of lights can be compared with the earlier experiences of Symeon. In his vision during the novitiate, he perceived first a sense of warmth, then a faint luminosity, a flash of lightning, and a flaming cloud. In later years, he saw the same, but the vision culminated in the sight of the sun, which absorbed the lesser lights and in which night and day became as one. He says, "It is a fire; it is a ray. It begins as a luminous cloud and ends as a sun."[15]

'Light' Symbolism in Symeon

"God is light" (I John 1:5); "I am the light of the world" (John 8:12); "You are the light of the world" (Matthew 5:14) were the three biblical verses that underlay Symeon's understanding of life in God. At the beginning he saw the light as formless and filling all space; later it began to assume a more definite 'shape', which he tried to describe in physical terms.

Symeon narrates a typical experience of his mature years: "As it willed, so it came, in the form of a shining cloud. It fell upon me, and I beheld it covering my head … Then I was aware of its presence totally within me, in my heart, and it looked like a shining orb, like the very face of the sun."[16]

Another narrative extends the astronomical metaphor: "What great wonder is this, hidden within me, of which I am aware but cannot grasp? Like a star, rising afar, it becomes like a sun, too great to be measured or weighed or defined. It rises a fine ray and then it blazes forth in my heart, deep within my body, whirling unceasingly, setting my body ablaze and turning it into light."[17]

This account suggests a twofold movement of the light: first, it appears at a distance, a mere point, and then it expands; second, the expansion of the light from star to solar sphere is at the same time its penetration deep into his embodied spirit, into the heart. Symeon emphasizes the supra-sensible nature of the light. It is totally other than the light of the oil lamp on his reading table, and even though it is said to be like the sun, it is an interior illumination that is totally other than the material light of the lamp and makes its flame seem a shadow.[18]

In one vision, Symeon hears the voice of Jesus: "I am the sun that rises each moment like a new day."[19] The rising sun, in Symeon's experience, is also the descent of the divine sun upon and within him. It is this descent that makes him ascend in the spirit.

The divine sun seems to shine from above, sending down a ray upon him, like a rope let down from heaven. He grasps the ray and flies upward toward the sun, but as he reaches it, he loses his grip and seems to fall back. The descent is at first painful and hard to accept, but he eventually realizes that his spiritual task consists precisely in this alternate ascent and descent, until he comes to the awareness of the non-difference between the rising and the falling phases. He says, "The beginning of the race is its end, and the end its beginning. Endless is its ending, for the beginning is already the end."[20]

The full moon in a clear night sky is an alternative symbol for the inner light (a familiar image of the contemplative state in tantric writings is that of the full moon reflected in still waters),[21] but Symeon does not develop the contrast between sun and moon. He does, however, describe his habitual state as one in which the difference between day and night disappears: "I see the light at all times, by night and by day; day seems like night to me, and night like day."[22]

'Fire' and 'Water' in Tantric Texts

The symbol of light evokes that of flame and fire, both in Symeon's writings and in the Tantras. By the practice of the yoga of 'heat' or *dumo*, Tibetan meditators seek to arouse the inner fire, identified with the vital energy that ascends from the base of the body's vertical axis. At the beginning of this practice, the passions (lust, hatred, envy, pride, and ignorance) emerge involuntarily, before they are burned away by the ascending flame.[23] Many Christian mystics have spoken in similar terms of their experience of 'passive purification', not produced by active, penitential practices but by the fire of divine love within them.[24]

In tantric experience, however, 'fire' is a symbol of union as well as purification. Abhinavagupta explains that, in the supreme intuition by 'divine means' (*śāmbhavopāya*), the yogi perceives the union of light in the human spirit as a 'consuming fire'.[25] His disciple Kshemaraja uses the familiar metaphor of iron in the forge to indicate the total transformation of the yogi in the fire of the divine *śakti*.[26]

All tantric yogis, whether Buddhist or Hindu, use 'fire' to indicate the union of the polar energies in the body ('sun and moon', *piṅgalā* and *iḍā*, 'white fluid' and 'red fluid'); these opposite forces converge and unite in the central channel or *suṣumnā-nāḍī* and rise upward as a single, golden flame. The fire flares up from the base of the spine to the crown of the head and permeates the entire body; the Tibetan yogis instruct us to visualize "the whole world as being permeated with fire in its true nature" and to cause the 'white fluid' (the 'male', cool current) to ascend from the base to the crown; then we are to make the 'red fluid' (the 'female', warm current) descend from crown to base, whence it flows through the entire body.[27]

In the 'lesser *kriyā*' or *haṁ-saḥ* practice described at the end of Chapter II, you accompany the first syllable (*haṁ*) by the thought of an ascending-white-cool-male current and the second (*saḥ*) by that of a descending-red-warm-female current. You can approximate the actual perception of coolness and warmth along the spine (an experience that is given to anyone who dedicates a certain amount of time to the practice) by slightly parting the lips ("as if to hold between them a long grain of rice," instructs Milarepa's disciple Gambopa). Do not purse the lips, as when you whistle or pronounce the vowels 'oh' or 'oo'. The breath must continue to flow through the nasal passages, even while it now passes also through the mouth; you feel the cool air flowing over your lips and tongue as you breathe in, and the warm breath as you breathe out. You will also hear the very soft sound of the primal vowel 'ə' (= 'a' as in 'was' or 'u' as in 'sun') in your breathing, without, of course, vocalizing the sound. Having experienced the coolness and warmth of the two breaths, interiorize this sensation and return to the mental recitation of *haṁ-saḥ* with lips closed. The identification of the incoming breath as 'male' and the outgoing as 'female' is a visualization process that focuses, not on the distinction of the two breaths, but on their union; as the terms themselves suggest, the two are to become one.

The symbol of fire, in all traditions, is closely linked to sacrifice. Abhinavagupta teaches that the heart is the unique place of sacrifice, both temple and altar. Gazing on the external fire of the tantric rite, the yogi unites this perception with the "fire of consciousness... deep in the heart." Abhinavagupta further instructs the yogi to "burn the body," that is, abandon the presumption that the Self is the body, and to offer the body to the Self; only in this way does the yogi become "perfectly stable, free of every disturbance."[28]

In Tibetan Tantrism, 'water', like fire, is also a unitive symbol. In the *Jetsün-Kahbum* (a 12th-century biography of Milarepa), it is said that two lights, "mother and offspring... inner and outer", become one in the great ocean of consciousness, the "illuminating-void awareness."[29] The *Mahānirvāṇa Tantra,* a Hindu text composed under Buddhist influence, sees the purificatory ritual with water as a bath in *tejas*, 'luminous fire'.[30] The process of purification, according to all these texts, has a moral dimension; it is not a question of eliminating ritual impurity but sin. This purification is effected by the ascending flame; at the summit of the bodily axis, the fire becomes 'nectar-like water' that washes over the burnt body and restores it to full integrity.[31]

'Fire' and 'Water' in Symeon

Symeon's mystical experience of Christ, as he narrates it, often begins with fire or a feeling of warmth, which then becomes light. The mystic's heart is a hearth or an altar, at whose center burns the fire of the Spirit; this burning produces both delight and suffering and generates intense desire for the divine vision. Symeon is wounded, inflamed, burned by the beauty of God, and yet, like the burning bush that Moses saw, he is not consumed. The flame is lit first in his mind, then in his heart, and thence it spreads throughout his being, transforming spirit, soul, and body. Like iron in the forge, taking on the nature of fire, the mystic takes on the nature of God.[32]

Transformation of spirit, soul, and body is closely linked to participation in the Eucharist.[33] Initiation into the Christ-life, like Isaiah's call to be a prophet (Isaiah chapter 6), requires that you 'eat fire', consume the flaming coal that the angel brings from the altar, so as to be pure in word, intention, and action. Symeon laments the unworthy ministers who act as if the sacrament in their hands were mere bread, when in reality it is fire.[34] But whoever is willing to be burned by the Bread and Cup soon beholds a great flame of divine love that raises the soul to the third heaven. Then the soul aflame is transformed into a fountain whose healing waters nourish the tree of life.[35]

In fact, water and fire express one and the same experience. Symeon speaks of both the eucharistic Cup and the Holy Spirit as a spring of living water; likewise, the incense used in the liturgical sacrifice is perceived by him as an inner unction, a water-source of eternal life, and a fragrant flame. Water is an especially dynamic symbol; Symeon says that the living water of the Holy Spirit illumines, inflames, and speaks. Even though the 'water of God' is an immense, unfathomable ocean, the mystic, possessing but a few drops of the water, partakes of the whole ocean.[36]

At first, Symeon's transformation by fire and water seemed to produce more smoke than flame, bringing to the surface all the dross of sin and passion; only when he was sufficiently purified did he begin to see himself in bright flames. One physical sign of the Holy Spirit's bath of burning water was the gift of tears. By means of tears, the painful searing of Symeon's early experiences was mitigated, and he felt cooled and refreshed.

He exclaimed, "The flame took hold and devoured me, and I was driven out of my mind. When I could stand it no more, tears gushed forth in an endless flood; this refreshed me and kindled an even more vehement fire, the fire of longing. From that moment tears flowed more and more freely; washed in their stream, I shone ever more brightly. At last, totally aflame and turned into light, I fulfilled [Christ's] saying, 'God unites with gods and is known by them'."[37]

The 'Five M's' in Tantrism

Against the 'old law' of the Vedas, Tantrism claimed freedom from the dichotomy of sacred and profane. According to the *Vijñānabhairava Tantra*, even the sense pleasures of eating, drinking, and aesthetic appreciation can lead to a high spiritual state. "The pleasures derived from music or through the senses of touch, taste, or smell can beget oneness of mind and peerless joy, by which the yogi becomes immune to ordinary pleasure and pain, and from such liberation of the mind can spring forth the flame of supreme bliss."[38]

The Tantra is not prescribing mere sense indulgence; what counts is the attitude or state of consciousness with which the yogi undergoes such sensory experiences. Eating, drinking, and listening to music become equivalent to sacred actions to the degree that one has realized the unity of the All in the divine consciousness. The fruit of a yogi's use of the senses is in effect like the passionless state sought by Christian ascetics: the yogi transcends the opposition between ordinary pleasure and pain and perceives the satisfaction of the senses from the viewpoint of supreme bliss.

Vedic rules of ritual purity can and must be rejected, when one has been purified by the practice of yoga. Says the *Vijñānabhairava Tantra*: "Bodily purity, as defined by those versed in religious lore, is but an impurity in the light of wisdom, and one who spurns all such distinctions between the pure and the impure attains real peace."[39]

Abhinavagupta also affirms that distinctions of pure and impure are not intrinsic qualities of things, like color, but are imaginary constructions. He affirms: "All is permitted and all is prohibited"; what makes the difference between yogis and mere libertines is that a yogi keeps the mind firmly fixed on the truth, and truth in all actions is the only inviolable rule.[40]

However much this doctrine may look like moral relativism, in fact the greatest purity, honesty, and selflessness have always been expected of yogis; what is really being said here is that the criterion of moral goodness cannot lie outside the person ('bodily purity') but must reside at the very center of consciousness or conscience ('truth in all actions'). It may be that Tantrism comes very close to Saint Augustine's famous paradox: "Love, and do what you will!"

The yogis' transcending of ritual purity and their engaging in profane activities entail the use of the *pañcatattva* or 'five M's': *madya*, wine; *māṁsa*, meat; *matsya*, fish; *mudrā*, parched grains; and *maithuna*, sexual union.

Traditional Brahmanism excluded all of these from ritual use as 'impure'; Tantrism introduced the five impure elements into worship in conscious polemic against the vedic priesthood. It is difficult to determine how these elements were historically used and what meaning was attached to them. Sexual union as a ritual action raises the question of 'sacred prostitution', so common in the ancient world; the prohibition of wine and meat was partly due to their supposedly aphrodisiac effects.

The question is ultimately whether and to what extent the substitution of vedic 'pure' rites with the 'impure' also entails interiorization, that is, whether the ritual use of the physical act or element is essential or whether drinking wine and uniting sexually are rather to be performed mentally as symbols of a higher reality. Some texts suggest that, in its earliest and most authentic forms, Tantrism understood the five M's as mental symbols and did not use them ritually (although it is a fact that Hindus living at higher altitudes, as in Nepal and Kashmir, do take meat and fermented beverages on occasion).

Yoga, conceived as a fire rite or sacrifice, implies transcendence and the 'rupture of planes', an ascent from the lower to the higher, from the exterior to the interior, from the multiple to the simple. Whatever the matter cast into the sacrificial flame, it is changed and transfigured; its nature and meaning are no longer the same. Even when the five M's are actually employed in ritual actions, their value for the yogi is always in direct proportion to their interiorization.

According to tantric teaching, there are three kinds of persons: *paśu* ('cattle' or 'carnal beings'), *vīra* ('heroic' or 'mental beings'), and *divya* ('divine' or 'spiritual beings'). Rules of ritual purity weigh heavily on carnal persons, who do not allow themselves to use any of the five elements as sacrificial offerings. Mental persons ('heroes') feel authorized to use them in a sacred context, in order to break the link between the elements and the purely sensual enjoyment of them. The spiritual person, the yogi, being truly free, has no need for the outward use of these elements; they are but symbols of what takes place interiorly.[41]

The references to wine and sexual union in the Tantras are understood by yogis as 'twilight language' (*sandhyābhāṣa*) or 'intentional discourse'.[42] Drunkenness and license in food and sex are symbols of specific stages in yogic experience, and the 'shocking' language of some texts serves as a mnemonic device to fix these experiences in the yogi's memory, as when they insist that *maithuna* is effective only when performed with a low-caste prostitute.[43] The *Kulārṇava Tantra* (5,111-112) makes clear the symbolic meaning: "The true *maithuna* is the union of the Parāśakti [*kuṇḍalinī*] with Ātman [Spirit, the Self]; other unions represent only carnal relations with women."[44]

In the last chapter of his *Tantrasāra*, Abhinavagupta explains the cultic practices of his school. Sacrifice, he says, can be offered in a variety of ways, only one of which is "exterior reality," but even in this case it must be performed while meditating on the essential unity of "breath, consciousness, and body" and while projecting the syllables of the *mantra* "on the head, the mouth, the heart, the genitals, and the whole body." The exterior rite can be begun without any preliminary purification other than "the meditative repose in the Self." Abhinavagupta devotes a long section of the chapter to *maithuna* but does not explain whether or not he considers this sexual union as anything other than a poetic metaphor for the union of *kuṇḍalinī* and Spirit, the male and female principles both interior and cosmic.[45]

The 'Banquet' and the 'Marriage' in Symeon's Poetry

One of the commonest symbols in the Bible and Christian tradition is the wedding banquet, the festive fulfillment of God's communion with humankind. Although the symbol refers primarily to the collective consummation of redeemed humanity in the kingdom of God, it is also understood as the personal union of the individual soul with the divine Bridegroom. This interpretation is already found in Origen's (third century CE) commentary on the Song of Songs, and Symeon the New Theologian follows this tradition.

However, there is something quite new in Symeon's treatment of banquet and nuptial symbolism. No other mystical poet insisted so strongly on the concrete reality of food and eros that underlies these terms. Symeon speaks from the experience of his own youthful debauchery when he proclaims the immeasurably more intense delights of the mystical union.[46] His language is almost crude at times, and one is reminded of the beat-generation poets. Yet the body does participate in the mystical experience, and the joy of the spirit overflows into the outer senses, fulfilling the yearning left unsatisfied in the passionate quest for pleasure.

The senses share in the joy of the spirit only when body and mind have been purified by the practice of active asceticism aiming at 'passionlessness' or the integration of spirit, soul, and flesh in the love of God.[47] The passions, habitual and often unconscious disorientations of our good appetites and energies, must be tamed and, in a symbolic sense, put to death, in order that our whole being, including the most refined emotions and sensibilities, may truly live. There is no philosophical hatred of the body in Symeon, but precisely because he loves his body, he cannot permit its forces to be scattered. He aims at 'one-pointedness' (*ekāgratā* in yogic terms, or 'purity of heart'), which focuses his entire being on the 'one thing necessary' and transforms his awareness of the All in the light of union with God.[48]

As we begin to focus our energies, we are aware of our own activity as distinct from what we understand as 'grace'. But gradually God's operations begin to effect a 'passive purification' of our nature, at times even in conflict with our ascetical activity. The mystical grace, although it is 'wine' for the human spirit, first works on us like poison, making us lose all taste for earthly pleasures.[49] But having reintegrated his humanity by ascetical practice and passive purification, Symeon speaks of his experience in terms of these very pleasures: he enters the bridal chamber; he lies upon the marriage bed; he eats fat meats; he drinks sweet wines![50]

The integrated, the 'pure of heart', are able to use their senses in a new way and with a new freedom. "To the pure all things are pure" (Titus 1:15); those who are capable of understanding fully their own natural impulses, who as it were 'dissect' the passions, are then able, like good doctors, to heal the wounded natures of others.[51] Symeon offers the example of his master as one who had overcome all false shame with regard to the body; he showed no embarrassment even if someone saw him naked.[52]

Symeon describes his freedom of body and senses with the metaphor of a connoisseur enjoying his first glass of wine after a long illness. He knows how to savor the delicate taste, because he drinks moderately, and he enjoys the color of the wine almost as much as its flavor and aroma. So entranced is he that he hesitates to drink, and yet the taste is so pleasant that he feels he could never be sated with it. The more he drinks, the greater his thirst.

The ray of sunlight shining through the glass has entered with the wine into his body and has transformed his members into fire. The wine, both nourishment and medicine, purifies his sick flesh and makes it whole, so that he has no taste for anything unwholesome. Healed, purified, and transformed, his whole body radiates the beauty and charm of an integrated human, "a friend of the sun and a beloved child of wine."[53]

The difficulty of choosing between the pleasure of the wine's color and that of its taste is indicative of the unity of the spiritual sense, which fuses into one all the various symbols: light, fire, water, wine, etc. The transformation of Symeon's whole being into light and fire by means of wine shows us the convergence of all the symbols in that of the 'heavenly nectar'. This intoxicating nectar or divine drink, inexpressibly sweet, flows from the breast of God; Christ himself is both mother and nurse, and his breast gives forth milk that is light.[54]

Symeon interprets very concretely, almost crudely, the apostle Paul's doctrine of the body of Christ and our union with him and one another as his members. Symeon compares spiritual teachers to the 'milk-giving breasts' and 'fertile loins' of a metaphorically androgynous Christ. These masters nourish God's beloved friends (the allusion is to the beloved disciple "lying close to the Lord's breast" at the last supper: John 13:23) with the food of angels ('heavenly nectar'), and they cast upon the soil of the disciples' hearts the fruitful seed of the Spirit. Symeon also applies this 'mystical anatomy' to the various virtues that make up our mature being in Christ; he even identifies the 'private parts' with "constant prayer and joy of the heart."[55]

Symeon makes his most audacious affirmation of our bodily union with Christ in *Hymn* 15, where he engages in an imagined argument with a fellow monk.

"If you are willing," he says, "you will become part of Christ, and all the parts of each one of us will, in the same way, become his, and he will become every part of us."

The listener looks troubled, and Symeon continues in more theological terms: "He becomes many, yet remains one, undivided, and each part is himself, the whole Christ." Then he reverts to the concrete, saying, "Since this is so, certainly you recognize Christ in me, in my finger, in my nuts!"

The listener blushes, and Symeon says, "Are you shocked? Why did you blush? God did not blush to become like you. And you, do you blush because you are like him?"

The other monk retorts: "No, that is not why I blushed, but when you said that he is like a shameful part of the body, I suspected you were uttering a blasphemy."

Symeon defends himself: "Wrong! You misunderstood; there is nothing shameful here. These are the hidden members of Christ, since we cover them, and by doing so, we honor them above the rest of the body, as the hidden members, which none may see, of him who is hidden."

Having bolstered his argument with the reference to Paul (I Corinthians 12:23-25), Symeon concludes his defense: "From him, when God unites with us, issues the God-formed seed, ah, the wonder! It is formed of God's own nature, totally his, for he is totally God. O awesome mystery! When he unites with us, it is truly a marriage, ineffable and divine!"[56]

This symbol of the marriage has various meanings in Symeon. Like many of his predecessors in the Greek church, he believed that, although God created the male-female polarity, the two were made to be one. Eve was originally in Adam; she and he were one being until she was taken from his flesh. When the humanity of Jesus was taken from the flesh of Mary, the order was reversed and the unity of the sexes was restored.[57]

Adam gave part of his flesh to Eve, and Christ now gives us his whole flesh in the Eucharist, taking each of us as his bride.[58] Christ's love for his spouse cannot be measured by human standards, for he has chosen as his own an adulterer and a murderer. Yet he loves her, and his mystical grace remakes her as a virgin.[59] This intuition of Symeon, grounded in the prophetic experience of Hosea (chapters 1-3) with his adulterous and meretricious wife, disproves the assertion of Mircea Eliade that, "from the Hindu point of view, the conjugal symbolism of Christian mysticism, in which Christ plays the part of the Bridegroom, does not sufficiently emphasize such an abandonment of all social and moral values as mystical love implies."[60] On the contrary, it is the very lack of 'respectability' in God's choice of lovers that is most often emphasized, both in the Bible and in patristic tradition, where the Church herself is sometimes referred to as *casta meretrix*, a 'holy harlot'!

---

1 EU 1,223-234; cf. H 45,32-39.

2 Cf. TE 3,160-171.

3 Cf. Vladimir Lossky, *The Vision of God*, pp. 91 and 117.

4 Cf., e.g., H 34,11-17; TE 5, *passim*.

5 Abhinavagupta, *Tantrāloka* 2,49 (Gnoli, p. 118).

6 Ibid., 5,86-95 (pp. 198-199).

7 *Mahānirvāṇa Tantra* 3,26 (p. 27).

8 *Tantrāloka* 5,47 (p. 194).

9 Cf. idem, 5,20-21 (p. 191).

10 Ibid., 4,89-91 (p. 165); cf. 5,22-25a (p. 191); 8,142a-146 (p. 260); *Mahānirvāṇa Tantra* 14,110-140 (pp. 347-351); *Shri-cakra-sambhāra Tantra*, p. 6.

11 Cf. Guenther, *The Life and Teachings of Naropa*, pp. 71 and 188.

12 Cf. idem, pp. 193-194; also Chang, *Songs of Milarepa*, pp. 47-48; 59; 206-207; Chang, *Teachings of Tibetan Yoga*, p. 39.

13 Cf. Guenther, *The Jewel Ornament of Liberation*, pp. 223-226 and 257-268.

14 Cf. Chang, *Songs*, pp. 156-157; *Teachings*, pp. 122-123; Guenther, *The Life and Teachings of Naropa*, pp. 60-61; cf. the 'signs of night' and the 'signs of day' in Chang, *Teachings*, p. 79; cf. also Evans-Wentz, *Tibetan Yoga and Secret Doctrines*, pp. 197-202.

15 H 17,325-327.

16 H 17, 373-387.

17 H 22,3-11.

18 Cf. H 25,5-20, and *Vie* 23,10 (Hausherr p. 33).

19 CT 34,334-335.

20 H 23, 401-414; cf. H 38, 93-100.

21 Cf. *Mahānirvāṇa Tantra* 14, 133 (p. 350), and Abhinavagupta, *Paramārthasāra* 7 (Silburn, p. 65).

22 H 18, 109-110; cf. H 17, 320.

23 Cf. Chang, *Teachings*, p. 78.

24 Cf. Symeon himself, in H 55,86-92; TE 1,12,209-221; CT 14, 83-94.

25 Abhinavagupta, *Tantrāloka* 3,285-286 (p. 152).

26 Cf. Kshemaraja's comment on *Spanda Sūtras* 6-7, cited in Silburn, *Hymnes de Abhinavagupta*, pp. 90-91.

27 Evans-Wentz, *Tibetan Yoga*, pp. 201-206; cf. also Chang, *Songs*, p. 157.

28 Abhinavagupta, *Tantrāloka*, chapter 13 (p. 212).

29 Cf. Evans-Wentz, *Tibet's Great Yogi Milarepa*, p. 152; Chang, *Teachings*, p. 30.

30 Cf. *Mahānirvāṇa Tantra*, 5,40-102 (pp. 66-77).

31 Ibid., p. 77.

32 These expressions are found throughout Symeon's *Hymns*; see especially 11,78; 18,98; 24,25-34; 28,140-190 and 150-156; 30,156-159 and 194-200; 30,426 and 488-496.

33 Cf. TE 1,10,55-75; H 20 passim.

34 Cf. H 58, 91-96.

35 Burning Eucharist: H 20,236-243; healing fountain: H 47,1-22; cf. the same symbolism in Maheshvarananda, *Mahārthamañjarī* 52 (Pereira, p. 386).

36 Cf. H 23,283-359; cf. also H 6,1-2; 17,519-624 and 831-832; 24,20; 28,129-131.

37 TGP 3,21 (third-person narrative rendered as first-person witness); Symeon quotes periphrastically John 10:34 (where Christ quotes Psalm 82:6), conflating it with John 10:27, hence the startling phrase, "God unites with gods and is known by them," which can, in turn, be compared with the tantric proverb, "Only a god can worship a god: *nādevo devam arcayet*"; cf. Eliade, *Yoga*, p. 208; Tucci, p. 29.

38 *Vijñānabhairava Tantra* 72-74 (Silburn, pp. 113-115); cf. Abhinavagupta, *Tantrāloka* 4,120-121 and 194-200 (pp. 168 and 177).

39 *Vijñānabhairava Tantra* 121 (p. 151).

40 Abhinavagupta, *Tantrāloka* 4,213b-221a (p. 179); cf. his *Tantrasāra*, p. 125.

41 Cf. John Woodroffe, *Tantra of the Great Liberation*, pp. cxi-cxx.

42 Cf. Eliade, *Yoga*, pp. 249-254.

43 Cf. idem, p. 261, note 204.

44 Ibid., p. 262.

45 Abhinavagupta, *Tantrasāra* 13, pp. 212-230, 277, and 281-298.

46 Cf. George Maloney, *The Mystic of Fire and Light*, pp. 23-24.

47 Cf. idem, pp. 112-154.

48 Cf. CT 31,90-115.

49 Cf. CT 23,9-11.

50 Cf. TE 6,115-129; H 46,30-39.

51 Cf. TE 6,249-278.

52 Cf. H 15,206-214.

53 CT 23,151-201.

54 Cf. H 50,143-152 and 28,183.

55 TE 4,369-514.

56 H 15,147-177.

57 Cf. TE 1,1,25-27 and 1,3,1-27.

58 Cf. TE 1,6,136-144.

59 Cf. TE 1,9,23-25.

60 Eliade, *Yoga*, p. 265.

Chapter V

The Ends of Yoga: Self-Realization and God-Consciousness

In the preceding pages, we have tried to sketch the lines of convergence between the symbolic language in Symeon's poetry and similar expressions in tantric texts. Their shared vocabulary of symbols is drawn from the human experience of this world's light, fire, eros, etc. The meaning of the symbols comes from faith; it is an understanding of the end already present in the beginning.

In every school of tantric yoga, the beginner, receiving initiation into *sādhana* from the guru by faith (*śraddhā*), receives an understanding of the way and its goal.

Faith in Tantrism is neither confidence nor belief nor intellectual assent taken singly, but rather a tension of the whole person who, by means of the creative imagination, seeks continually to verify the content of faith by experiencing it or by becoming it. This is not the empirical verification demanded by natural science; it is a personal realization that transforms one's total existence as body, soul, and spirit.

By faith, the human self is realized as the image of what is contemplated, and contemplation consists in seeing through the image into the full light of Reality shining beyond it. By faith the disciple embraces spiritual authority, whether this is seen in the sacred texts, in a lineage of teachers, or in an interior, guiding illumination. Yogis submit to this authority, because they see in it the light of its transcendent origin and its ultimate end. Faith is *śraddhā,* that is, yogis 'put' (*-dhā*) their 'heart' (*śrad-* or *hṛd-*) into the hands of the guru, because they are convinced that a beginner's effort is already a participation in the perfect end.

A similar concept of the act and habit of faith underlies Symeon's narration of his mystical experiences. He began as an orthodox believer, but the link between his belief and his first visions of the light was not immediately apparent. It was only by faith in his spiritual father, the elder Symeon, and by the faith in Christ that both received from the Church, that he came to see the Christ of faith in the light and fire that rose up within him. At the same time, the experience transformed his faith and brought it to maturity. Symeon recognized God in the light, and what was initially only an overwhelming experience became a personal encounter.

Symeon often used the negative or 'apophatic' language typical of Eastern Christian mysticism: the light is formless ("a form without form"), and the sight of it is beyond expression in human concepts and words. Given the abyss of difference between God and myself, I can speak of God only in negative terms, because any experience of God is incomprehensible, ungraspable, incommunicable. When I see God in this life, I am seeing "in a mirror, darkly," as Saint Paul said (I Corinthians 13:12).[1]

Yet Symeon also insisted that the mystical graces he received were a conscious experience. Transformed and illumined by the vision of light and fire, Symeon's spirit reflected, in its undivided attention, the unity of the Godhead, perfect, simple, unchanging. His vision of the one light was equally a vision of the three: aware that he was using human words to express what is essentially inexpressible, he said that the Trinity appeared to him like a radiant face with two shining eyes: these are the Son and the Spirit, proceeding eternally from the Father.[2]

The personal energy of the Holy Spirit reveals God to us as light.[3] If the trinitarian light seems abstract when reduced to the poverty of human words, then a better word for the light of the Spirit is love. This love is one and indivisible; it is the same charity that is the life of the faith community, binding the people of God together in holy fellowship. The personal illumination of a mystic is always ordered to the building of what Symeon calls "the city of love," in which all are one, and God is all in all.[4]

The process of illumination begins with what Symeon calls "baptism in the Holy Spirit."[5] Symeon does not use this expression in opposition to sacramental baptism in the Church as body of Christ; he is speaking of the dynamism of the sacrament itself, which tends toward an ever-expanding consciousness of the indwelling Spirit. Many 'mere Christians' are content to live unconsciously; they refuse the personal experience of God and stifle the Spirit. For Symeon, they may as well not have been baptized.

The Holy Spirit gives us a foretaste of the spiritual and corporeal union with Christ that we hope to enjoy in the resurrection. The Holy Spirit 'spiritualizes' our bodies through the struggle for holiness in this life, until they shine in the full fire and light of God.[6]

Symeon focuses on the embodiment of the eternal Son of God in Jesus; he meditates on the mystery of the divine Word becoming flesh in the womb of the Virgin Mary, then dying on the cross and rising to become mystically embodied in the Church. From his Christ-centered meditation Symeon develops a theological anthropology or *physiologia*, a doctrine of human nature in the concrete order of grace and salvation history.[7]

Jesus Christ, the *Logos* enfleshed, is the image and likeness of God, and we are made "according to" this image (Genesis 1:26); Christ is the second Adam, the new human who came "in the likeness of sinful flesh" (Romans 8:3) in order to restore what had been lost by the first humans (Genesis 3:1-19). Symeon understood this restoration in the most concrete sense possible, repeating the great axiom of Saint Irenaeus: "God became human so that every human being might become God." Our 'divinization' (*theōsis*) is not confined to the soul but extends to body and senses. In the vision of light we are made light; by grace we rise with Christ.

One of Symeon's favorite gospel verses was "Blessed are the pure of heart, for they shall see God" (Matthew 5:8). He understood the two clauses of the beatitude in close and reciprocal connection; the purification of our whole nature as spirit, soul, and body is both the condition and the effect of our vision of the Christ-light. Symeon identified blessedness with the unitive vision of God, and this vision is a dynamic and continuous process that begins in this life and leads to the blessedness of eternal life.[8]

There are conditions, of course, for beginning this mystical process and arriving at the eternal glory that is its end. We must willingly participate in the sufferings of Christ, in order to share his resurrection. We do this by patiently bearing the ills of this life, by practicing the physical and spiritual methods of asceticism, and by receiving Christ in the Eucharist. Symeon's whole life and doctrine were centered on faith in Christ made really present under the species of bread and wine, food and medicine for soul and body.[9]

We can trace two dimensions in the meaning that Symeon discovered in his experience. The first is a personal meeting and union with God in Christ and the Holy Spirit. Symeon recognized, by means of faith, the person of Christ in the light and fire that rose up within him. Heaven was opened, and he saw God. But he also says that what he saw was an outward manifestation, the "glory of God", and that it was the "eye of the heart" or his mind that was opened. This is the second dimension of Symeon's experience: the consciousness of his own transformation by light and fire.

Whether we consider the light as 'God-consciousness' or as 'self-realization', in reality it is one and the same. Our transformation into God is our vision of God; we were made to see God in our own transfigured spirit. These expressions may sound 'pantheistic'; Western theology has acquired an almost pathological fear of such expressions, but in doing so it has tended to make Christians forget a very important aspect of biblical and patristic teaching. "Whoever is united to the Lord becomes one spirit with him" (I Corinthians 6:17); my awareness of being transformed by grace and my awareness of God's presence in me are 'one consciousness'.

Transformation of Consciousness

In Symeon's writings as in the Tantras, 'consciousness' is a dominant concept. The symbol of light implies an opening-out, leading to the awareness of the true self, of reality, of God. Yoga can be defined broadly as 'transformation of consciousness'.[10] This is not necessarily a 'consciousness-of'; yoga brings human consciousness to the realization of itself in an activity that is totally free from limiting conditions because it is totally free from objects other than the very act of consciousness. In other words, yoga can be described as a continuum of consciousness that is light and union, rather than a consciousness of light or union. This means that the yogic state or activity (they are the same thing), being free from the otherness of objects, can also regard objects, but in a different way.

The highest consciousness to which the yogi aspires is not emptiness of the mind but a transformation of mind and thought that radically changes the mind's relation to its contents. This datum of experience cannot be explained directly; it can only be suggested by symbols, such as light, fire, and mystical marriage.

Some yogis, especially in the Hindu devotional tradition, have experienced transformation of consciousness as a gift or 'divine grace'. Far from seeking to absorb the object of devotion, these yogis realized the self in abandonment to a higher Self, whose personal nature transcends even the Absolute, Nirvāṇa, or Brahman. They know the true self by self-giving, in a play of uniting that never ends, for there is no suppression of the two who are made one in love. This understanding guided Paramahansa Yogananda's practice and teaching of yoga. Now as we describe the outward practice, we set our hearts upon a twofold intention: to seek consciousness of God by offering our consciousness to God.

What Yogananda called Kriya Yoga and identified as a true 'fire rite' was called *yajña* by his guru, Swami Śrī Yukteśwar.[11] This term properly identifies the bloodless rites and sacrifices that only brahmins may perform. The yogic *yajña*, given freely and openly to humanity without mediation through hereditary priesthood or ritual practice, makes of every human body a temple and every human spirit a priest. Its "principal requisite," says Yukteśwar, is "the heart's natural love." The practice I describe here differs in various ways from the *kriyā* transmitted by Yogananda's disciples and codified in their printed lessons; it represents an alternative initiation to which I have had access.

You have by now become accustomed to identifying the incoming breath with an ascending, male, cool current along the body's vertical axis and the outgoing breath with a descending, warm, female current. You have also experimented with slightly opening your lips, so that the breath flows gently, in an uninterrupted cycle, through both the mouth and the nasal passages. The gentle breath, without any action of the vocal cords, creates the sound ə (the 'a' in 'was' or the 'u' in 'sun'). The yogic *yajña* (the 'greater *kriyā*') now requires that your breathing become much deeper, while remaining steady and slow, with no holding of the breath at any point in the cycle. You will find that, with the outgoing breath, the back of the tongue will naturally rise toward the soft palate, shaping the oral cavity so as to produce a breathing-sound rather like the 'i' in the word 'is'.

No vocal sound is to be made; the breath itself, inhaled through the nose and slightly-parted lips, produces the vowel sounds 'a' (*uh*) and 'i' (*ih*). These sounds produced by deep breathing must be audible to yourself and anyone sitting close to you. It is not necessary to maintain the mental recitation of *haṁ-saḥ* as you breathe.

The incoming breath should take from nine to eighteen seconds (begin with the shorter timing and gradually extend it). Do not hold the breath in, but pass without interruption to the outgoing breath; the out-breath should take the same amount of time as the in-breath and should not be held out. The two breaths constitute a single cycle or act of *yajña*, with a duration of eighteen to thirty-six seconds. Perform no more than twelve of these cycles in any given meditation period, and then return to the normal *haṁ-saḥ* breathing, with lips closed. When this yogic sacrifice has become a part of your daily life, you may gradually increase the number of cycles.

The value of yoga lies not in psycho-physical procedures but in the sacrificial intention and heartfelt devotion with which you perform them. In the *Yoga Sūtras* of Patañjali (2,1), physical practice (*tapas*) and study of sacred teachings (*svādhyāya*) culminate in the yogi's total abandonment to the Lord (*Īśvara-praṇidhāna*). Self-surrender and self-forgetfulness are the conditions for becoming conscious of your true self, which you will find only in God.

The 'Fourth State' of Consciousness and the Goal of Yoga

We have seen, in the tantric way of perfection, the three factors that are, at one and the same time, limits that bind us to the profane condition and the necessary instruments for passing beyond that condition: embodiment in the flesh, the world, and time. The goal of the tantric yogis was not to eliminate this threefold embodiment but rather to find transcendence, the consciousness of their native freedom, within human life, *mukti* within the condition of *jīva*.

Tantrism's concept of transcendence through integration is rooted in a common scheme of Indian metaphysical thought: that of 'the three and the fourth'. In Western philosophy, two opposing poles are transcended by a third; Hegel expressed this basic logic, derived from the Greeks, in his dialectic of thesis-antithesis-synthesis. Indian logic and metaphysics posit three terms in an immanent dialectic and a fourth term that transcends the three.

Prakṛti, Nature, is characterized by the three qualities or *guṇas* (*tamas*, *rajas*, and *sattva*, sometimes translated 'inertia, energy, and harmony') and is transcended by Spirit, *Puruṣa*, which is *nirguṇa*, 'without qualities'. In human life, the three psychological states of waking, dreaming, and dreamless sleep are transcended in the 'fourth state', which is often identified with the high-point of yogic meditation, *samādhi*. In Patañjali's yoga, posture, breath-control, and sense-withdrawal, the three practices grounded in the body and the senses, are preparatory to, and transcended by, *saṁyama*, Patañjali's collective term for the three practices of the one-pointed mind: contemplation, communion, and assimilation (*dhāraṇā*, *dhyāna*, and *samādhi*).

Tantrism, especially the school of Abhinavagupta, applies this scheme to all levels of reality: the being of God, the energies of the cosmos, and the inner life of the soul.[12] The yogis of Kashmir follow the psychological doctrine stated in the *Śiva Sūtras*: the 'fourth' is not another state differing in degree or kind from the three (waking, dreaming, and sleeping) but is the transcendent dimension of consciousness present within the three.[13] This immanence of the fourth in the ordinary states of consciousness has important consequences for the practice of yoga. We have already examined, in chapter II, the dialectical relationship between 'practice' and 'realization', that is, between yoga as effort and yoga as the recognition of the non-difference between bondage and liberation. This dialectic does not, of course, eliminate the skillful use of means in yoga, but it does relativize all means in view of the end. The three means enumerated by the Kashmiri yogis, the particular, the energic, and the divine, correspond to the three *śaktis* or energies by which the transcendent deity self-manifests in the universe, the *śaktis* of activity, consciousness, and will. God is one being with the *śaktis*; likewise the goal of yoga, the highest consciousness, is already present in the means. The beginner's initial effort, understood as 'grace' or a descent of divine energy (*śaktipata*), is already God-realization.[14]

Yogis who practice particular means like breath-control or sacrificial rites are predominantly aware of their own effort and of distinctions between means and end, between their own consciousness and God. The energic way involves a progressive purification of the differentiated consciousness (*vikalpa*), which, in the initial stages of *samādhi*, is still aware of the knowing and the known as distinct from the knower. The divine way is union and freedom, through knowing the known in the knower and the beloved in the lover; it is the immediate intuition of God through God's image in the soul. This is *nirvikalpa samādhi*, identified with the fourth or transcendent consciousness.[15]

Abhinavagupta also speaks of a yogic consciousness that can be called 'trans-fourth' (*turyātīta*), a state beyond *samādhi* that is none other than the blessedness of the Lord himself and thus is a means that is 'no-means' (*anupāya*). At this level, there is no longer the 'I' of the yogi who 'realizes God'; the yogi's 'I' is simply God. This, for Abhinavagupta, is the ultimate grace: "The domain of the heart, that of the Supreme who comprehends the All within himself, is spontaneously realized by the person upon whom falls the grace of the Lord, and effort no longer plays any part."[16] Yoga is no longer a practice separated from life, but every movement of the body is a *mudrā* or yogic gesture, every word on the yogi's lips is a *mantra*, and every breath is *prāṇāyāma*. All is grace; all is yoga; God is All.

Tantric yoga's conception of the goal, the highest state of consciousness, is 'evolutionary'; consciousness is, in fact, *spanda*, vibration, a continually evolving reality. In Kashmiri Tantrism, the light of consciousness is indissolubly one with its energies, the power and activity of thought. It is not a detached 'witness', untouched by multiplicity and becoming; it is an act, just as God is the infinite act, the 'vibration' at an infinite frequency that brings the universe out of nothingness and animates its every movement.[17] The ultimate end of the yogi is a paradoxical one-pointedness that is experienced as an uninterrupted expansion of consciousness, a conscious participation in the omnipresence of God.

The Degrees of Contemplative Consciousness

How might Symeon have described this yoga of the transformation of consciousness by grace? When he speaks about the 'consciousness of grace', he is in effect describing a 'grace of consciousness', the gift of a new way of knowing, in which God is known in the mutual opening-out of 'heaven' and the 'mind'.[18]

Only when I accept grace as such, that is, as God's free self-giving and not as a 'thing' or 'created quality' in the soul, do I become conscious of God, who is no longer a concept in my mind or an object outside of me. God takes my mind, my thinking, my awareness, and changes the way they relate to persons and objects in this world. I become aware of God, when God acts upon me to make me 'become God', to assimilate me to the divine likeness; it is this likeness that is both my true self and my consciousness of God. This new consciousness is not a psychological 'act' or 'state'. It is not caused by an 'object', because God is not an object I think about but a living presence within me. The effect of God's self-giving is a deep change, a newness in the human spirit itself.[19]

Symeon affirms that the true Christian is the person who possesses Christ consciously, "in fact and by experience, by the senses, by knowledge, and by contemplation."[20] Underlying this affirmation is the ancient doctrine of the three stages in the spiritual life: *praxis* (moral-ascetical practice), *gnōsis* (knowledge or contemplation of nature), and *theologia* (contemplation of God).

In this life we often experience the flesh as a burden on the soul, but in fact, it is the soul's disordered activity, not the body, that leads to sin and the darkening of the divine likeness in us. The practice of moral and ascetical virtues purifies the senses and emotions from passionate attachment to creatures and awakens the soul's capacity to see them in the light of God.[21] This knowledge of created reality is completed by the contemplation of the divine light.[22] The person who attains this *gnōsis* sees God in all things, and the ascent through creation culminates in a vision of the mystery of God, both benign and fearsome.[23]

In a teaching to his fellow monks, Symeon describes this ultimate stage: "If you cling to God and know God by practice, you will be deemed worthy to see God with your whole being by contemplation. But what you see I could never write down. Your spirit beholds strange wonders; you are wholly illumined and become luminous but are unable to think or speak about all this."

Symeon continues his description of the progress through communion with God's light to assimilation to it as a turning inward alternating with expanding consciousness: "You see yourself wholly united to the light, but as you concentrate upon the vision of yourself, you return to your former state. As you grasp the light within your soul, you enter into a state of ecstasy, and in this state you see the light as if from afar. But once you have returned to the center, you find the light again." Symeon admits that he is completely at a loss for words and concepts; he finds it hard to tell about or even to understand what he sees.[24]

Categories of 'within' and 'without', of 'self' and 'other' cannot be applied except paradoxically to this state. Symeon's very self seems to be the light, a luminous source that illumines all things; yet he is conscious of having received the light as a grace given through faith. Although his vision is a single, indivisible act, it is not without a dynamic movement of contraction and expansion. When the experience begins to have effects on his psyche and its faculties, Symeon reflects on these psychological reactions, goes into ecstasy, and the light recedes. But when he turns back from attention to self, he discovers the light once again, shining brightly in the center of his heart.

The 'formless form' of the light is beyond all conceptualization; likewise there is no way of saying whether consciousness is focused within or expanded outward to the infinite. It is one with God's light, whose center is everywhere and whose circumference is nowhere.

The Meaning of 'Higher Consciousness'

From yogic sources we can discern three stages in the evolution of consciousness. In the beginning, one makes use of definite objects, whether physically present or imagined, and the subject is aware of the distinction of knower, knowing, and known. By the progressive abstraction of the objects, the knowing subject itself is 'abstracted', that is, drawn away from the object and turned in upon its own activity of knowing. This serves to purify the yogi's spirit to the point that the course of thought is stopped, fluctuations cease, and the spirit beholds its own natural light. This is the stage of *kaivalya*, 'isolation', of which Patañjali speaks: a contemplation paradoxically full and yet devoid of objects. Centered in itself, the yogi's spirit is out of all things: the body, the world, the flux of time.

Abhinavagupta, however, and the tradition he represents, insists that this stage is not the final one, precisely because it is an altered state and is bound up with certain psychological conditions and with the practice of meditation as a distinct activity. The ultimate stage of yoga, for Abhinavagupta, is the mystical union with the Lord. The Supreme One is not a detached and static 'witness' but a living person mysteriously hidden and revealed in the three energies of will, consciousness, and activity, and in the many beings of the universe, which form God's 'body' or outward manifestation. In the same way, the perfected yogi hides and manifests the awareness of this union in the activities of everyday life, in artistic creation, in the performance of religious rites, etc.[25]

On the psychological level, there is no passing back and forth from a mystical to a profane consciousness; the light shines through every thought and feeling. Says Abhinavagupta, "Thus awakened by the stimulus of the mystical realization, the yogi sacrifices all psychological distinctions (*vikalpa*) in the luminous flame of the Self and becomes one with the light."[26] Although yoga as practice requires concentration, the focusing inward of consciousness on the indivisible point of light, the Self, once the yogi realizes the Lord in the Self, the light radiates outward in a continuous expansion of consciousness, filling the universe as the Lord does.

Symeon uses the same language to describe his experience of the final stage of mystical union: "From this stage, you are in the light, or rather united with the light, but not as if you were in a continual state of ecstasy. Rather you perceive yourself, your surroundings, and your neighbor as they are… because here and now the light dwells in you and makes you light."[27]

The way to this higher consciousness of God begins with applying the mind to particular objects, which may be both sacred and profane. I contemplate the virtues of the many beings on earth and in the wider cosmos, and I interiorize these virtues in the course of meditation. This contemplation of nature has two functions: to discern the glimmers of God's light in creatures, which imperfectly mirror God; and to train my spirit to see its own light, to behold within itself the very image and likeness of God. This light is mine by 'nature', because it is of the nature of my spirit to be open to God's free self-gift in grace.

When Symeon first beheld the natural light of the mind, the divine form impressed upon his human spirit, he was in an altered state, both ecstatic and one-pointed. His whole being was centered, concentrated on the light, and taken out of the world of objects and even, it seemed, out of his body. He was conscious of the light, without being able to form concepts about it, since his being was totally centered in the faculty of mystical cognition.[28] He was at a loss to explain the light, even in terms of his faith. But this one-pointed ecstasy, his spirit's vision of its own light, indistinguishable from the light of God, was a state that stopped the course of thought and blocked the activity of the psyche, and for this reason was not yet the full mystical vision.

The ultimate degree of consciousness, the goal of the mystical quest, is not itself an altered or extraordinary state; it is rather the natural state of the human spirit, transformed into the light that is God. When the spirit reaches this level, it begins to free the mental faculties to assume once more their proper functions, while remaining in the light. The soul is no longer carried out of itself but begins to live in the habitual awareness of a luminous presence. As the light becomes more familiar, its links with the understanding of faith are re-established, and the mind discerns in the experience itself the meaning given by faith.[29]

One final point needs to be clarified. The highest consciousness that mystics attain, whatever their faith tradition may say, seems to be of a non-dual nature. This fact has created difficulties for what is said to be the dualism that underlies traditional Christian metaphysics. How is this dilemma to be resolved? Perhaps one way out of it is to note the widely differing metaphysical notions of non-duality found in the various Hindu and Buddhist schools. For instance, Abhinavagupta's non-dualism is different from both Vedantist and Buddhist monism, in which the One is precisely a 'state', a static reality, while for Abhinavagupta it is *spanda* or movement, vibration, energy; hence, you could say, his 'One' is many!

Christian orthodoxy need not deny what so many Christian mystics affirmed: that they were 'annihilated' in God, that in them God knew God, God saw God, and their very 'I' was God. From Saint Irenaeus, who said, "God became human so that every human being might become God," to Saint Catherine of Genoa, who said, "My 'me' is God, and no other 'me' do I know," there is an unbroken golden thread of mystical doctrine. But mysticism is not metaphysics, and the One of the mystics is not a state of their consciousness. Their experience is rather a continually self-transcending movement into the One God, a movement that begins in this life and will continue for all eternity.

---

1 Cf. TGP 2,18-19 and CT 16,135-139.

2 Cf. H 12,23-24 and TE 8,99-123.

3 Cf. CT 14,102-141; TE 6,140-145; and H 25,36-46.

4 Cf. H 32,3-28 and CT 1.

5 Cf. TGP 1,35-36 and 3,43-45; cf. also CT 2,251-261 and 32,79-86.

6 Cf. TE 7,513-517.

7 Cf. TE 1 passim.

8 Cf. TE10,778-867.

9 Cf. H 19 passim.

10 Such a definition does not, of course, exclude transformation of the body; cf. Bede Griffiths, *Return to the Center*, p. 136.

11 Cf. Yukteśwar, *Kaivalya Darśanam: The Holy Science* (Los Angeles: SRF, 1972), pp. 33-65.

12 Cf. Kanti Chandra Pandey, *Abhinavagupta: An Historical and Philosophical Study* (Varanasi: Chowkhamba Sanskrit Series, 1963), pp. 597-604; Lilian Silburn, *Le Paraamārthasāra*, pp. 20-26.

13 Cf. *Śiva Sūtras* 1,7 and 3,20 (Gnoli, *Testi dello Śaivismo*, pp. 38 and 44).

14 Cf. idem, 1,5 (p. 37).

15 Cf. Silburn, *Le Vijñāna Bhairava*, pp. 20, 33-34, 40-41, 94-95.

16 Abhinavagupta, *Iśvara-pratyabhjñā-vimarśinī*, vol. I, p. 7, line 14, cited in Silburn. *La Mahārthamañjarī*, p. 15.

17 Cf. Silburn, op. cit., pp. 22-42, and Gnoli, *essenza dei Tantra*, pp. 29-33.

18 Cf. Maloney, *Mystic of Fire and Light*, pp. 11-14 and 58-63.

19 Cf. Anselm Stolz, *Teologia della mistica* (Brescia: Morcelliana, 1947), pp. 148-151 and 160-163.

20 CT 8,28-29.

21 Cf. H 4,35-51.

22 Cf. TE 6,219; H 21,400-439.

23 Cf. H 38, 84-92.

24 CT 2,353-364 (second person discourse as dynamic equivalent of his third-person rhetoric).

25 Cf. Abhinavagupta, *Iśvara-pratyabhjñā-vimarśinī*, I,6,7 (in Silburn, *Le Paramārthasāra*, p. 53, note 4).

26 Abhinavagupta, *Paramārthasāra* 68 (p. 85).

27 TE 1,12,433-442.

28 Cf. TGP 2,16-18.

29 Cf. TE 1,12,351-451; H 27,96-118; H 51,18-63; EU 2,132-146.

Chapter VI

The Process of Yoga: The Ascent of the Inner Fire

The goal of yoga is 'transformation of consciousness'; I experience it as a grace by which my spirit assumes the form of God as light. But I am not just spirit; I am also psyche and flesh. I am a being whose essential dimensions are spirit, soul, and body, the integration of which is part of my spiritual goal.

The personal energy of the Holy Spirit, a divine 'fourth dimension', begins to penetrate into the three dimensions of my nature, and at first I feel more strongly the distinction and even the tension and conflict among them, fruit of the disorder of sin.[1] This is the 'purgative' phase of the spiritual evolution. To the degree that I grow in the light (the 'illuminative' phase), I see the dimensions of my nature come together. In the end, when their original unity has been restored (the 'unitive' phase}, the light will enable my body and mental faculties to share in the transformation of the spirit, without taking me out of the normal condition of life.[2]

My body becomes divine in union with the divinized body of Christ. This union is a gift and a promise for humanity as a whole, and each individual shares in the divine body by uniting with all others in the 'mystical body', whose efficacious sign is the Church, sacrament of the incarnate Son and temple of the Holy Spirit. Symeon takes this doctrine literally; for him, each participant in the sacramental mysteries becomes a member of Christ's body, and every part of his or her physical body becomes a member of Christ.

The body purified and divinized through contact with the sacramental Body in the Eucharist. This purification is passive, an operation or energy of the Holy Spirit, but it is also active, the fruit of striving for a 'passionless' state, in which natural energies are ordered toward the 'one thing necessary'. Active purification is paradoxical, for by quieting disordered desires I become a "man of desires" (Daniel 10:11 in Greek) and experience the reintegration and transformation of body and psyche as an embrace of love.[3]

The light of God shines in the transformed spirit, but it also shines in the flesh. In one of his most impassioned hymns, Symeon sings, "What measureless compassion is yours, O Savior!… Your own body, immaculate and divine, is totally resplendent with the light of your Godhead, with which it is ineffably mingled and made one. And all this you have given to me as well, O my God!… I am made one with your Godhead and am become your own immaculate body, a brilliant member, a truly holy member, from which and through which your brightness shines."[4] But as Symeon exults in his transformation, he never forgets that, absent God's grace, his body remains a "filthy and decaying tent," and he himself is "unclean and a wastrel and a rake." But Christ chooses prostitutes, rakes, and sinners as his lovers.

The flesh, made transparent to the divine light, is transformed when Christ raises it up from the mud, touches its wounds, and heals it. But as I receive this work of grace, I must also work on the active purification of my body. Symeon saw the ascetical and devotional disciplines of his tradition as removers of impediments to the light, much as tantric yogis see postures and breath control as preparatory to the awakening of *kuṇḍalinī*. More important than external exercises is the 'energic way', and so we ask how the awakening of a potential energy in the body might be related to what Symeon and his tradition say about the role of the flesh in the spirit's illumination.

The Evolution of Energy According to the Tantras

Tantric yogis observe within the body various points where the conscious spirit seems to come to a focus; these points are oriented along the body's vertical axis, centered in the spinal column and meditatively conceived as the 'center of the world'. The energy that brings the cosmos into manifestation and the energy that gives life to the flesh are experienced as one fire, which ascends through the centers of consciousness along the body's axis and links the flesh to human and divine consciousness.

There are some obvious similarities between Symeon's narration of his experiences and what the tantric yogis say about the awakening and ascent of *kuṇḍalinī*. Of course, what is similar may not be identical; I am only speaking in terms of an analogy of experience. I hope to show how a Christian who has this kind of experience (whether he or she arrives at it by using some yoga exercises or simply by the Jesus prayer or other Christian method) will find in it a meaning that corresponds to his or her faith, much as Symeon did in the course of his illumination.

The energy of which the Tantras speak is of divine origin but assumes many forms, in both the cosmos and the body. Within the body, this energy exists in a potential condition, 'folded in' upon itself; human evolution, the transformation of consciousness, depends on its 'unfolding' until it becomes 'straight'.[5] Hindu texts personify the energy as a *śakti* and depict it as a serpent coiled at the base of the spine. Buddhist Tantras do not use this symbolism for the vital energy of the cosmos and the human body, but Buddhist and Hindu texts alike conceive of it as a force lying at the base of the body's vertical axis, in proximity to the organs of generation; in the practice of yoga, the force ascends to the summit.[6]

In addition to being 'folded in', the energy is also dispersed horizontally throughout the various organs and functions of the body. The yogi works to draw these forces together into their original unity and redirect them up and down through the various centers of consciousness, until they come to rest as one divine energy in the center of the heart.

The concentration and elevation of the energy within is accomplished principally by means of intense mental focus, aided and made efficacious by the control of breathing. Even a brief practice of the basic *haṁ-saḥ* breath-cycle demonstrates to the practitioner how closely linked are breathing and thought. This link is intensified in the act of breath-*yajña* described in chapter V, but the ultimate result of this *prāṇāyāma* is not greater tension and need for control but a return to the slow, natural pattern of breathing, in which the in-breath is accompanied only by the sense of wonder and the out-breath by the sense of delight.

However, the elevation of the vital energy is an arduous task and involves moments of real tension between the ordinary 'downward' or 'in-curving' tendency of this energy and the yogi's efforts to 'straighten' and 'elevate' it. The awakening of the *śakti* leads to the 'piercing' and 'burning up' of the centers of consciousness in the body (*cakras*), and as the metaphors suggest, this cannot take place without pain.

The yogi's task is not only to elevate the energy but also to allow it to descend. The practice of breath-*yajña* involves precisely this alternate raising and lowering; only after the fire has consumed all the centers does it come to rest in the heart, and the yogi feels the body is being showered with cool, celestial waters or 'ambrosia'. The beginner senses that the central channel, the *suṣumnā-nāḍī*, is 'tied in knots', and great effort is required in order to untie it. At the same time, however, yogis experience the arousal and ascent of the vital energy as a grace, a descent of the divine energy upon and within them, and this experience ultimately dominates their efforts and enables them to transcend the external practices of breath- and thought-control.

Divine Grace and the 'Evolutionary Potential'

Mystical experience is always an experience of unity, both one's inner unity and union with God, the transcendent Absolute. As an experience, it is also conscious, indeed a new consciousness. As I sought this unity, I accepted the following premise, which I found was affirmed by all Christian mystics and many tantric yogis: that union with God does not destroy human nature, enfleshed in the universe and in time, nor is it a fusion or confusion of the human person with the divine Being. This same premise underlies even the 'monistic' or non-dual language that mystics use.

As they struggle to express their experience, they acknowledge the mysterious antinomy of God, who really self-manifests and really makes us "sharers in the divine nature" (II Peter 1:4), while remaining always God, "beyond every name and every essence" (John of Damascus). The Infinite God remains God, and the human person "becomes one with the Infinite without any loss of individuality," as Śri Yukteśwar taught.[7] God and the human are made one in love by the grace of God, who is the Giver of all gifts.

We are wrestling with the mystery of God's freedom: God creates and loves us and showers upon us the divine All. The self-giving of God in love is grace. Grace is thus an 'energy' of God, rather than a 'thing'. Our deification by grace must be understood in terms of two affirmations, which are related as an antinomy: grace must be 'mine' (otherwise it is not my deification), and grace must be 'divine' (otherwise it does not deify at all).

From the Bible, Christianity draws the teaching of the temporality of creation, in both its origin and its subsistence. The world began at a given moment (the beginning of time) and remains in existence at every moment of time in virtue of the creative act of God.[8] Creation is not, even metaphorically, a 'design'; it is a simple, unceasing, free act. To call God an 'intelligent designer' contradicts both the transcendence and immanence of God, who is rather the Mind (metaphorically speaking, of course) in whom all things exist eternally and by whom all things have existence in time, at every instant.

Man and woman were made "according to the image and likeness of God" (Genesis 1:26-27). The original image is the eternal Son, made flesh in time as Jesus Son of Mary; by grace we grow in this image and assume an ever more perfect likeness to incarnate Godhead. Eastern Christian thinkers have always emphasized the unity of the natural order and that of grace, seeing our participation in God in a dynamic perspective. We are by nature open, evolving beings, and grace is a challenge. We are called to grow, and we are given the power to participate actively in effecting this growth.

Each of us is, by nature, a microcosm: human nature unites in itself something of all the various creatures (we possess life in common with plants, senses in common with animals, spirit in common with angels). By union with God, the human person unites the various polarities and conflicting forces of created being and brings the whole world to its unity in God. However, in the concrete order of things, the human being is, as Symeon says, a 'double being', a composition of opposites and a living contradiction. The other polarities in the world are rendered more acute and irreconcilable by the divisions within our own being.[9]

Through the incarnation of God in Jesus Christ, these divisions are ultimately reconciled. Symeon calls him the 'double God', who constitutes the unity of microcosm and macrocosm and above all the unity of God and creation.[10] The Incarnation restores unity in a fractured world, but even absent the 'Fall' (cf. Genesis 3:1-13), the Word would have become flesh as the culmination of creation's evolution and return to God.

The basis for our deification, says Symeon, is the union of God with our human nature in Christ. We understand this union of divinity and humanity in one Person by our own participation in it.[11] We share in 'Christhood' by grace, and our union with God has a 'Christic' quality. The human flesh of Jesus, consubstantial with ours, is the cause of our deification, because our human nature was deified in him. While they subsist only in his divine Person, the natural functions ('energies') of the human dimension are neither suppressed nor deformed. The humanity of Jesus is not made less human, but it is deified by the divine energies; the operations or influences of divinity transform the flesh, mind, and will of the Savior into perfect instruments of God's will.

God's Uncreated Energies

Following Symeon, the Eastern Church gradually elaborated a doctrine to aid in understanding, within limits, the mystery of our union with God. This is the doctrine of the 'uncreated energies' that proceed from the divine essence but are not identical with it.[12] They are not creatures; in ultimate analysis, they are less 'things' than 'activities'; indeed the Greek *energeiai* is correctly translated 'operations' in many texts. The energies are God in contact with, and permeating, the created universe and especially its sentient beings. The energies are the three Persons of the Trinity in their loving, personal, 'outward' self-manifestation.

Since union with God is a dynamic process continually in act, both the innate dynamism of human nature and the movement toward participation in God that we call grace are the work of the uncreated energies. Keep in mind the concept of these energies as 'movement', as we try to relate this teaching to the *śaktis* and especially *kuṇḍalinī* as described by the yogis.

The energies are, first of all, uncreated. They would proceed from the Trinity as an aureole of glory even were there no creation. Their reality and their distinctness from God's essence do not depend on the existence of a world. But the world's existence and evolution are, in fact, the temporal manifestation of God's eternal energies. The universe, this planet, our psycho-physical activity, our evolutionary potential are truly operations of God, whose personal involvement in all this makes creation real. Created beings do not produce the uncreated energies; on the contrary, they are produced by the energies, and thus the creature's being and operations manifest God's personal and operative presence in creation.

On the basis of this teaching, let me advance the following hypothesis: the ascent of the fire within me and the effort I exert in order to awaken it are part of the movement toward deification that is both the evolutionary dynamism of nature and the operation of God's grace. The psycho-physiological factors in this movement manifest the activity of the divine energies; they reflect by nature, and act in harmony with, the uncreated energies of God.

Considered abstractly, human nature does not require divine grace in order to evolve into what it is meant to be. But in the concrete order of 'graced nature', evolution both biological and spiritual is effected by the synergy or unity-in-action of God's energies and nature's potential. Synergy implies freedom, and this means that individual human beings can and do refuse to evolve, to flow with the current of the uncreated and created energies, which tend toward the union of all in God. But aside from the possibility of individual failure, human evolution is one movement in which both human and divine operations are united, without mixture or confusion, and with the pre-eminence and freedom of the divine activity.

The conception and birth of the eternal Son in Mary's womb is an example of the activity of God's energies in a biological function. Applying the analogy of the incarnation to our spiritual evolution, we can say that, when we receive the Holy Spirit, God's energies are made manifest in our biological and psychological functions, especially our understanding and free will. God is present in these functions, directing them toward our perfection, which is conscious union with God. We consent, collaborate, and carry within ourselves the 'seed' of the energies, but the 'fruit' that is born of this union is a divine reality, that is, the transformation of our consciousness by grace, toward the likeness of Christ.

In order to clarify this hypothesis, we can use three metaphors suggested by the mystics of the Eastern Church. The first is that of 'reflection'. The uncreated energies 'reflect' the divine essence from which they proceed, as in a spotless mirror; by receiving the energies, we truly possess the light of God. Likewise, the image of God in us, as a work of the uncreated energies, is like a mirror; the energies operate in us to render it spotless, that we too may reflect God's glory. The creature's movement toward God in love is a reflection of God's love and movement toward the creature.

Another metaphor is that of 'sympathetic vibration'. The uncreated energies strike a responsive chord in us, in our senses and biological life as well as in our spirit, much as a note played by a violin can cause a piano string, tuned to the same pitch, to vibrate without being struck. In other words, our created energies are 'tuned to the pitch' of God's energies.

Finally, we can speak of the manifestation of uncreated energies in us as "the lamp of the body"[13] (called the 'single eye' in Matthew

6:22, King James version). This lamp is lit by the flame of God the Holy Spirit, operating through uncreated energies. Once the lamp is lit, the flame is a dimension of my total life, and I am responsible to see that its light is never extinguished.

The Awakening and Ascent of the Inner Fire

Jesus reveals a transfigured humanity; in him the divine and human energies are indivisibly united, and all the forces of his humanity are integrated and oriented toward the operative manifestation of the divine Person, the Word. Gazing on him, I see what my own humanity is destined to become. Union with the deified flesh of the Savior is both the end and means of my practice, even though, as means, it may be distinguished as 'particular', 'energic', and 'divine'. As 'energic means', union by grace with the humanity of Jesus is a process of focusing and elevating the energies in me.

For some persons, the awakening of fire occurs suddenly and unexpectedly, as it did to the young Symeon. In my case, thanks to the practice of Kriya Yoga, the process assumed a slow tempo, and the experience came upon me subtly and gradually. At first I felt a faint warmth along the spinal axis, then felt it concentrated in the head, and flowing into the heart and other members of the body. A light was there, beyond the darkness of closed eyes, without form, vibrating in many colors.

Yogananda and his guru taught their disciples to expect a sound to arise in their meditation, like the piano string resonating without being struck. The sound is an echo of the divine energy that vibrates throughout the universe. I first discovered this 'cosmic *oṁ*' while standing in an empty auditorium at night, a few months after Kriya Yoga initiation. From then on it has been present in meditation, as 'the sound of silence', a 'white noise' like that of the froth on ocean waves or the wind sighing through pine needles. I hear it only if I attend to it; otherwise, it is not there, nor does it disturb my normal hearing.

A skeptic may suggest a prosaic explanation for these phenomena. It is not necessary to claim anything supernatural about them. God's energies work unobserved, in and through natural energies, and arouse in the beginner an expectancy that will stimulate the effort to practice.

Like Symeon as a novice, I meditated on the lives of the saints, and this awakened in me the expectation of one day beholding, as they did, the glory of the Lord. I dwelled on what the saints must have felt and what their attitudes must have been, when the light dawned upon them: joy, a sense of unworthiness, wonder above all. At the same time, I engaged in the effort to open my being to God's energies. Breathing practices focused my will to raise up the life within me toward the divine presence, which is in the depths and at the center of my being, and indeed fills the whole universe.

The consciousness of the end (expectation) and the will to attain it (effort) do not contradict the gratuity of divine grace. God is a totally free giver, and God's greatest gift to the creature is a progressively greater freedom, a share in the very liberty of God. When the divine energy awakens within me, I begin to realize how truly unworthy I am of such an experience, which is not something I achieve but is God's gift, to which I must not and cannot cling.

It is only when I touch the depths of detachment that the power flashes through me like lightning, descends into my bowels as a consuming fire, and rises within me like a great flame, lifting me up with it. This power effects a process of painful cleansing. At first, it brings to the surface all my suppressed desires and passions and makes my present state seem worse than before. The effectiveness of my efforts begins to wane, and I slowly learn to yield to the energies of God that flow through me. As the knots of my nature are untied, my wounds are healed, and gradually the forces dispersed in the passions come together again.

Ultimately, the polarity and conflict of flesh and spirit will be reconciled, and the double being that I am by nature will become one in itself, as I become one with the double God, the incarnate Word. Then the consuming fire will have become a cooling water that refreshes and washes my burnt flesh.

Likewise the apparent duality of grace and effort will disappear; the inner light will be a second nature. The various centers of consciousness in the body (forehead, throat, heart, navel, genital) and all its members will become equally luminous; having seen the light of God in a part, I shall see it in the whole. I shall realize that in my beginning was my end, and that end and beginning are one. When time is permeated with eternity, the here and now become a foretaste of the ever-new and everlasting joy.

Desire and Love in the Awakening of the Inner Fire

No theological language is perfectly adequate; it always falls short of the mystery. Perhaps you could say that the model of 'energy' applied to God's self-giving in grace is inadequate on account of the apparent impersonality of the term, especially as it resonates with technological connotations, such as electrical and atomic energy etc. But in the writings of the Eastern Church mystics, the term has a profoundly personal significance. The energies are God, the Trinity operating freely and lovingly through creatures.

In considering yoga as practice and realization, I have yet to speak more fully about the 'way of love' (*bhakti-mārga*) in those schools of Tantrism to which Yogananda and his gurus paid homage. The yogi's striving is not a cold, calculating manipulation of faceless forces but rather the longing for mystical union. Devotion to the Lord and to the *śaktis* that emanate from the transcendent nature is the fundamental and indispensable practice of yoga for Abhinavagupta and his school.[14]

The goal of tantric yoga is a mystical marriage. This symbol alone should suffice to indicate the personalism of both means and end. For a Christian, too, the effort to raise up the energy within, through practice, is a reaching-out to a Person. The light, when it first appears to me, does not clearly reveal its 'who' or 'what', but eventually I see it, by faith, hope, and love, as Christ made known in the gift of the Holy Spirit. This gift is bestowed on all who seek to be united nuptially with the Lord, so as to bear him in their body and become "one spirit with him" (I Corinthians 6:17). This union is all the more profound because Lover and Beloved remain two in essence though one in love;

what individuality remains is only such as is necessary and sufficient to say, "I love you," for all eternity.

The light that flashes through the body, that rises like a sun in the heart, sets the soul aflame with desire for God. This desire grows all the more intense as phases of light alternate with darkness, expansion with contraction. Eventually the desire itself prevails and becomes light, dispelling the shadows of personal suffering and resistance to grace.

As love grows, it exposes ever more clearly my sinful inconsistency with God's gift.[15] Desire is both joy and pain, scorching flame and cooling dew. The gift of tears is an outward, visible sign of, and a sharing in, the process of purification effected by the divine energies. My striving to raise the energies, to stir up the grace within me, to ascend from the depths of my divided and wounded nature, is a constant process of 'conversion', *metanoia*, which is both penitence for sin and a 'change of heart', a transformation of the spirit that becomes once again the limpid mirror in which the clear light of God is reflected. This change of heart, a gift of divine mercy, the return to the center, the homeward journey of the prodigal child, is a discovery of the 'center everywhere' of God's love, an encounter halfway down the road with the Father running to meet me, showering me with signs of his love (Luke 15:11-32).[16]

This return to the center is the discovery of the nuptial chamber, the secret place in my spirit where I am embraced by the Lord and receive a new life, a seed that will grow for all eternity. The experience is also like a feast, and when the fire has reached the summit and center, it flows forth as wine, intoxicating me with joy. I do not cling to the wine and joy as if they were mine alone; I have them only because I am in the Bride, to whom alone they belong. I am but a cell of the Cosmic Mother whom John the Divine saw, clothed with the sun, crowned with twelve stars, and with the moon under her feet (Revelation 12:1). She is the *ekklēsia*, and being catholic, she is virtually all of humanity, indeed all life. As a contemplative, said Symeon, I am her fruitful loins, her breasts; when I teach, I cast the divine seed into others and assist at their birth. This is my yoga, the yoga of the heart.[17] Having found my heart, I know that it is one with the Mother's heart, and hers is one with God's.

---

1 Cf. H 55,86-114; TE 1,12,209-221; CT 14,83-94.

2 Cf. H44,147-165; TE 1,3,99-119.

3 Cf. H 9,16-39.

4 H 2,1-22.

5 Cf. *Vijñānabhairava Tantra* 154 (Silburn, p. 168).

6 Cf. Anagarika Govinda, pp. 139 and 193.

7 Yogananda, p. 490.

8 Cf. John Meyendorff, *Byzantine Theology*, pp. 133-143.

9 Cf. H 13,18-30; H 23,72-79; H 31,133-141; H 53,101-131.

10 Cf. H 25,62-66 and H 32,92-103.

11 Cf. Meyendorff, pp. 159-165.

12 Cf. Meyendorff, pp. 185-189; Lossky, *Mystical Theology*, pp. 67-90.

13 Cf. H30,78-160; CT 33,1-79.

14 Cf. Lilian Silburn, *Etudes sur le Śivaisme du Kaṣmir*, Tome I: *La Bhakti* (Paris: Boccard, 1964).

15 I hesitated to use the term 'sinful' here; the Greek *harmartia* suggests another metaphor: 'sinning' means 'missing the mark'.

16 Cf. H 17,715-738; H 24,42-62; H 56,18-20.

17 On 'heart yoga', cf., in general, *Le Coeur*, Etudes Carmélitaines 29 (Bruges: Desclée de Brouwer, 1950), pp. 88-95; also Silburn, *La Mahārthamañjarī*, pp. 25-26; 50-54; 95-100.

Chapter VII

The Means of Yoga and the Practice of Meditation

If yoga is the way of the heart, of grace and love, what then of 'techniques'? Said a monk-artist on Mount Athos, "Technique can never produce a true icon." If the icon of Jesus in our soul is ultimately the work of God the Holy Spirit, then our nature and all our efforts are but the medium in which she works. And yet the individual soul is an artist in her own right.

Tantrism also sees a tension between yoga as practice and yoga as realization or 'recognition' of the actual union between particular consciousness (the human individual) and absolute consciousness. Schools that consider *bhakti* (what Śri Yukteśwar called "the heart's natural love") to be the chief practice of yoga relativize all other efforts of the individual, while teaching the necessity of breath-control, meditation, etc.

Ultimately we come to the simplest definition of yoga, that given by Patañjali in *Yoga Sūtras* 1,2: "Yoga means stopping the agitations of the heart."[1] Note well: 'stopping'. Yoga is as much about *viyoga*, 'unyoking' or 'undoing', if you will, as it is about control or discipline or technique. When you have gone beyond curiosity and superficial enthusiasm, you realize the need to 'stop' and 'undo' and 'unmake', if you are to get anywhere with yoga.

Yoga practice aims to stop the agitations of the heart, not so much to 'control thoughts'. 'Distractions' in meditation are there for a reason: to reveal what is just below the surface of our minds, that which we do not observe because we are indeed distracted by the much ado of our lives. Distractions do not break the intention, and both prayer and yoga are all about intention: why do you pray? (not: what are you praying for?); why do you meditate? The answer of the Tantras is: to be free. Traditional Hinduism posits 'liberation', *mokṣa* or *mukti* as the great end, and it seems that, for most people, this means being set free from the trammels of body and world. The goal in the Tantras is recast as *svātantrya*, 'liberty' rather than 'liberation'; and if *mukti* is spoken of, it is with reference to the ideal of the *jīvanmukta*: the person who is 'freed while living' in the body and the world.

The phases of yoga in which human activity predominates are 'particular means', *āṇavopāya*.[2] They are the means proper to the 'individual' (*aṇu*, literally 'atom'), but even these are under the aegis of the *kriyā-śakti* or 'energy of activity', and from the beginning they are dominated by the fundamental attitude of the yogi: wonder. For the *Śiva Sūtras*, "All the stages of yoga are wonder."[3]

Not-Doing and Doing in the Yoga Sūtras

Patañjali enumerates his own series of stages, the eight 'members' of yoga practice. The first two (*yama* and *niyama*, 2,30-32) contain five words each; they are about the yogi's general intentions and behavior. Although they are commonly seen as a kind of 'ten commandments', and the two 'tables' (*yama*, *niyama*) are translated as 'prohibitions and precepts', they are more descriptive than prescriptive, and their meaning can be grasped only as a whole.

The first of the ten words governs all of them: *ahiṁsa*, 'harmlessness'. Like the first precept of the Hippocratic oath (*Primum non nocēre*) it means that yoga practice must do no harm either to the yogi or to others. Pushing through pain in performing postures, extending meditation periods beyond an hour, holding the breath more than three or four seconds: all these introduce a tone of violence into yoga and are contrary to the authentic sacrificial intention, which is one of yielding, offering-up, abandonment, surrender.

Gentleness and harmlessness govern the yogi's use of speech. *Satyam*, truthfulness, does not mean saying out loud in every circumstance what you regard as true. It means a silent demeanor that renders the yogi's right conscience evident and gently corrects wrongdoing by the contagion of example. Truth means never judging. The only negative precept of Jesus was: "Judge not." In the intention of Jesus, this rule is absolute and universal, because we can never know what is in the heart of a person. Jesus knew, and he said, "Father, forgive them, for they know not what they do." Truth in our minds also entails our recognition of how little we know and our sincere willingness to learn.

Asteya, "Not to steal," means never to take what was not given freely. Many yogis, like Buddhist monks, are mendicants, but they are not active beggars. If they have needs, they leave a bowl at their side while they meditate. Yogis with family and social responsibilities practice scrupulous honesty in all their affairs and would rather not acquire goods than to harm someone by acquiring them; the rule is always harmlessness, *ahiṁsa*. All yogis practice gratefulness, and they know that what is enjoyed without giving thanks is as if it were stolen.

Prohibitions about sex are an obsessive distraction in most religious teaching. The fourth word in Patañjali's decalogue, *brahmacarya* (literally, 'journeying in the Absolute'), is a positive term. It expresses primarily the yogi's commitment to integrating the body's energies into the spiritual quest; a secondary meaning of the word is 'chastity'. Properly speaking, chastity is a virtue of lovers; its practice is the intimate sexual relationship between two persons dedicated to each other. Even yogis who have no partners practice this virtue as if they loved someone dearly enough to do absolutely nothing to harm the relationship; the governing principle is *ahiṁsa*, harmlessness and non-violence. In practice, neither self-pleasuring nor physical intimacy in a faithful relationship are impediments to the practice of yoga or the search for God. I have found, in my personal experience and through many years of counseling others, that emotional and psychosexual maturity are attained as one's sex life is purified of violence, obsessive-compulsive behavior, and false guilt. Psychological counseling may be in order, but both personal sexuality and deep yoga meditation facilitate this process.[4]

The last negative word in the *YS* 2,30 is *aparigrahā*, which means something like non-grasping; it corresponds more or less with the tenth commandment of Moses, "Do not covet." It could also indicate a willingness not to cling to persons or things, because doing so would be a form of violence and so run counter to *ahiṁsa*. In all cases, we need to see through the grammatical negative in ethical teaching and observe the positive virtues: the life-giving and healing act, the comforting and enlightening word, the generous gift, the tender and loving embrace, and a general lightness of touch that respects the integrity of persons and things: these are qualities that yogis strive for.

Ahiṁsa overflows into the other five words (*niyama,* YS 2,32), which are grammatically positive. *Śauca* means 'cleanliness' and is practiced by yogis as frequent bathing and regular bowel habits, etc. Contemporary society has totally secularized this part of life, and that is good. Tantric yogis keep themselves clean but do not give value to what traditionally is considered 'ritual purity', another obsessive religious distraction. Jesus, by his explicit teaching and personal example, abolished the received rules about 'clean' or 'impure', whether regarding foods or persons.

'Contentment', *santoṣa*, is another positive expression of the precept of *ahiṁsa*, which governs a yogi's whole existence. The concrete meaning of *santoṣa* can be updated in terms of contemporary 'green' concerns; the 'slow' movement (slow food, slow fashion, etc.) and the theme of 'elected simplicity' also show today's need for the recovery of this yogic virtue.

The final three words have already been given in the first verse of *YS* 2, with the name of *kriyā-yoga*. This literary inclusion suggests that these three words are a governing principle for all ten, like *ahiṁsa*, They are *tapas*, literally, 'fervor', or technically, 'corporeal asceticism'; *svādhyāya*, 'study of one's own [tradition, teachings, scriptures]'; and *Īśvara-praṇidhāna*, 'abandonment to the Lord'. These three terms imply a tripartite anthropology of body, mind, and spirit. *Tapas* can be understood to include all three 'outer members' of

Patañjali's system, that is, *āsana*, 'posture'; *prāṇāyāma*, 'breath control'; and *pratyāhāra*, 'sense withdrawal'.

Of course, *ahiṁsa* rules here as well, especially with regard to the postures: the only instruction given by Patañjali is that the body should be steady and comfortable. In other words, the yogi assumes a meditation posture that allows the mind to remain focused and awake. *Prāṇāyāma* is not about 'control' so much as about breathing according to the non-violent and self-surrendering intention of 'harmlessness' and 'abandonment to the Lord'. For this reason, the true breath-sacrifice does not require forced holding-in; occasional suspension of breathing or "ecstatic apnea" will happen spontaneously after regular and protracted practice of the lesser and greater *kriyās* (see above, chapters II and V). Moments of this breath-ecstasy have been given me, especially in India, and then slow and relaxed breathing resumed. Finally, sense-withdrawal follows the same criteria of harmlessness and abandonment and consists mainly in the observation of sensory experience without forming judgments in the mind. The quiet and dimly lit environment appropriate to meditation will limit sensory input, so that the meditator can discern the fragmentary and transitory nature of all sensing.

Tantric Rites

The particular means of tantric yoga are not exclusively the corporeal techniques of hatha yoga or even the 'eight members' of Patañjali's system. Tantrism also elaborated a system of rites, initiatory and sacrificial ceremonies, as substitutes for the official rites of temple Hinduism.[5] Tantric ceremonies, as opposed to vedic, do not usually have a secret or exclusively sacerdotal character, and they are more directly joined to the practice of yoga.

The Tantras unanimously insist on the interiorization of the rites; the goal of 'higher consciousness' excludes a purely material or magical role of body, gestures, and objects in tantric ritual.[6] This is not to say, of course, that no tantric schools ever tended in that direction;

such aberrations have occurred in the history of Christian spirituality as well.

Tantrism interiorizes cultic symbolism in two ways: by investing the psychophysical practices of yoga with ritual value, and by 'projecting' ritual acts and objects on the body. The first method follows in the line of a long-standing tradition already present in the Upanishads and highly developed in the *Bhagavad-Gītā*. This key theme is Tantrism's closest link with the religion of the Vedas; in fact, tantric writings often simply repeat the expressions and ideas of the Upanishads and the *Gītā* concerning interior worship.

The *Vijñānabhairava Tantra* gives great importance to the understanding of yoga as the most perfect form of worship. Having described the yogi's goal as union with the divine consciousness, the Tantra poses a metaphysical dilemma: since the worshipper and the deity are now one, how can there be any exchange of gifts between them?

In a concluding dialogue, the disciple asks a rhetorical question of her teacher: "Of what use is offering oblations to the sacred fire, and to whom is a sacrifice to be offered?"

The teacher answers, "Time and again it is in the supreme Self that contemplation becomes absorbed, and in that blessed state the recitation of prayers is spontaneously maintained through the uncaused sound."[7]

The sound referred to is the 'cosmic *oṁ*' perceived inwardly as a sign of ascending *kuṇḍalinī*. This sound is manifested in speech, and as the *Śiva Sūtras* affirm, every word a yogi utters is a prayer, not only the sacred formulas of worship.[8] It is not by imagining the various forms of divinity but by maintaining the mind still and like a spotless mirror, that the yogi enters into the meditative state. Perseverance in this state is the only true worship.

Says the Tantra, "Worship does not consist of merely offering flowers. When the intellect is grounded in the highest void bereft of all ideas, that is real worship, conferring utter tranquility based on faith."[9]

The flower offering is important in *pūjā* or tantric sacrifice, but the only 'satisfaction' or fruit of ritual works that the yogi seeks is the 'unlimited fullness' of consciousness. In the words of the Tantra: "Into the fire of the supreme void the yogi casts all beings, the organs of the body, and external objects, for the highest form of offering is that in which the mind is the sacrificial vessel."[10]

The yogi rejects the ulterior motive that vitiates all ritual worship: the obtaining of 'satisfaction' and favors from God in this life and the next. Practicing the tantric way of "destroying all bonds and harboring all things," that is, simultaneously but on different levels renouncing and embracing every kind of human experience, whether worship, food, sex, or the arts, the yogi worships in that "sacred space where Lover and Beloved are one."[11] Only on this condition do worship and the fruits thereof lead to liberation.

This is the 'sacrificial intention' in which the different planes of yoga meditation and ritual intersect and ultimately merge. The 'particular means' of ritual and breath-control are swallowed up in the 'energic means', and the only *mantra* is the automatic repetition of *haṁ-saḥ* as the breath flows in and out naturally. But even this comes to an end in the 'divine means' of total assimilation to the Ultimate (*nirvikalpa samādhi*), when, having drunk the 'supreme ambrosia' more precious than life itself, the yogi is lost in the embrace of the Beloved with her Lover.[12]

So far we have seen the first mode of interior worship according to the Tantras: yogic practices and meditative states are given ritual meaning and value, thus fulfilling religious demands for offering worship. The other mode, the meditative interiorization of ritual acts and objects, is no less important. The two basic forms of tantric worship, initiation and sacrifice, are closely united. Each initiatory rite culminates in the act of offering, and sacrifice itself is conceived as a continual initiation, inasmuch as it is a progressive penetration of the yogi's understanding into the spiritual meaning of the rite. The matter of the offerings is normally 'unbloody': water, the camphor flame, incense, and flowers; these represent 'sacramentally' both the material cosmos (the elements of water, fire, air, and ether) and the worshiper's body (the successive *cakras* or centers of consciousness, from the genital level up to the forehead). These same offerings have been integrated into the Christian Eucharist at the ashram of Shantivanam in South India.

Two key elements in tantric ritual constitute a bridge between the outer form and the interiorized meaning: *mantra* and *maṇḍala*. *Mantra*, as a 'tool of the mind', is the instrument for the rupture of planes between action and thought, between exteriority and interiority. Every ritual formula, whatever may be its literal, 'gross' meaning, always refers to a 'subtle' reality, whether an aspect of the divinity, a point in the yogi's body, or a state of consciousness. The tantric worshiper must keep in mind both meanings, in order to perform the rite validly. Ultimately, the need for the gross rite is overcome, and only the subtle, spontaneous repetition of the *mantra* remains, linked with the breath.

The *maṇḍala*, the tantric icon, is also an instrument for placing ritual objects (the offering or the divinity itself) on the subtle plane, within the yogi's body. In its outer form, the *maṇḍala* takes the place of the vedic altar and is thus already a spiritualization of the rite. The *maṇḍala*'s form also suggests a 'march toward the center', a rite of initiation in which the adept progresses through various levels to reach the inner sanctum of the *bindu*, the indivisible point that no longer has any meaning except on the level of yogic consciousness, where it paradoxically becomes an infinitely expanding circumference.

The process of interiorization does not by any means exclude the divinity itself, the object of worship. In Buddhist Tantrism, the various gods and goddesses are invested with ritual but not ontological value, until they are revealed as nothing other than symbols that efficaciously evoke particular states of consciousness in the yogi. In the end, worship is understood as being offered solely to the luminous void of the Buddha-mind, completely realized in the mind of the yogi. The Hindu yogi also realizes the self in the Self, but the One whose essence is consciousness transcends and embraces both unity and multiplicity. On the level of experience, the yogis do not eliminate *bhakti*, devotion to the divine Person, upon attaining Self-realization and union with the Ultimate.

Interiorization of Worship in Christian Meditation

The interiorization or inner projection of cosmic and cultic symbolism is central to tantric yoga and is intimately connected with such practices as posture and breath-control; this may be called the 'soul' of yoga practice. The interiorization of the mysteries of the gospel are also a necessary task in the spiritual life of a Christian meditator. However, the total absorption of the rite into meditation raises questions for us, given the centrality of the historical incarnation of God as seen by Christian faith.

The most helpful insight that Tantrism offers us is the way it resolves the tension between the sacred and the profane by the positive and sacrificial value it gives to all human experience. Christianity, too, proclaims that "To the pure all things are pure" (Titus 1:15), but the concept of 'sacramentality' means more than this; it implies a real continuity between the 'everyday' and the 'liturgical', between body and spirit, between earth and heaven.

Interiorization, in the sense in which Symeon and other Christian mystics understood it, can be accomplished only through a profoundly personal experience of the God who is effectively present in the world, as well as in the sacramental signs (water, bread, wine, oil) drawn from this world. God purifies, sanctifies, and deifies the participant in the sacraments through physical contact with these signs, which are thus called 'efficacious' in virtue of the Holy Spirit's descent into their materiality. "Only a god can worship a god" is a saying of the tantric yogis; Symeon said, "God unites with gods and is known by them." The progressive deification of the human being by grace is the necessary condition for a sacrifice that is both interior and sacramental.

In virtue of Christ's sacrifice in a given moment of history, and in virtue of our participation in this sacrifice through its real presence in the eucharistic bread and wine, we are empowered to offer "spiritual sacrifices acceptable to God" (I Peter 2:5). The spiritualization that the Bible proposes does not eliminate the external expression of worship but rather grounds it in human nature, which is both 'spiritual' and 'bodily'.

The apostle Paul said, ""Present your bodies as a living sacrifice, holy and acceptable to God, which is your spiritual worship" (Romans 12:1). Just as Christ is the abiding sacrifice in the Eucharist, so in him we are a living sacrifice, and all our life assumes a cultic value. Of course, the individual's participation in the church's worship is not always, and certainly not automatically, interiorized; the spiritualization of the Christian sacrifice requires constant effort.

While I receive with joy the Christ who comes through consecrated bread and wine into my heart, I also feel the need for an evolution of my consciousness, in order to realize more fully his presence in me, in the sacramental signs, and in the community of faith that celebrates Christ's presence. My task is to discover both the external sign's meaning and its internal effect in the Christ whom I meet in my meditation and in the activities and relationships of my everyday life.

The soul of all tantric exercises, whether postures, breath-control, or ritual acts, is the mental projection of cosmic and ritual symbols upon the body and especially upon the centers of consciousness (*cakras*). This method renders bodily practices efficacious in awakening the dormant vital energy.

Patañjali's expression, *kriyā-yoga*, is often used in tantric literature to denote union (*yoga*) by means of a sacred activity (*kriyā*) that has many levels of meaning. First, it means the active movement of breath: the yogi aims not so much at stopping the physiological process as at breaking its links with time, eliminating the irregularity of its rhythm, slowing it, and conceiving each breath as a total cosmic cycle, a day and a night or even a year or more. The second level of meaning in *kriyā* is the movement of energy, the ascent and descent of fire along the spinal axis, which is the true *prāṇāyāma* or control of vital energy. The third level is the consciousness of the movements of breath and the inner fire as a sacrificial activity, a fire-rite in which the yogi's being is consumed and given over wholly to God. At the first level, the subject of the activity seems to be solely oneself, but on the other two levels the yogi perceives the activity of the Spirit as predominant; God's Breath breathes in the yogi's breath. For the Hindu yogi, no less than for the Christian, 'activity' without 'grace' is sterile.

Cosmos and History

The yogis of Hindu and Buddhist Tantrism realize the whole cosmos within their bodies: the body's vertical axis is the center of the world, around which revolve the sun, the stars, and the entire zodiac, until they fuse in the center, where the hub and the rim of the universal wheel are one. Christians have inherited from the Bible a different world-view, grounded in the understanding of time as history. An early Christian teacher, Irenaeus (second century CE), saw Christ as the point in which cosmos and history converge; Christ 'recapitulates' both. In Irenaeus' vision, history is not only linear but is also a 'Christ-ring' that unites beginning and end, creation and eternal glory, in the incarnate Word. This vision of unity is the center of Christian meditation.

Symeon the New Theologian presents his own method of interiorization in Hymns 18 through 20, which form a single poem. He begins to relive the whole history of the Bible as a consequence of the inner light, which, upon its arrival, "took possession of my head." The flame, now stirred up, "reaches the heavens"; it is in heaven, but it is also in Symeon's heart. The light, unrecognizable at first, now illumines his understanding of the mysteries of faith: "It reveals the Scriptures to me and increases my knowledge; it teaches me mysteries that I cannot express."

When Symeon encountered his master, the elder Symeon, he was like Israel in Egypt, a slave and a stranger. The old monk, appearing in Symeon's first vision of the divine light, is at first like the angel that Moses saw in the burning bush; later he is like Moses himself, summoning Symeon from slavery. Symeon goes forth from his spiritual Egypt, but the journey is not easy; Pharaoh, the power that enslaved him, pursues him into the desert. But the young man is victorious over his enemy, having been "turned into light" by the prayers of his master.

In the next stage, Symeon comes to recognize the face of Christ in the light; Symeon realizes that he enjoys a greater grace than did Moses of old, having "seen the face of the Lord," who is none other than the Eucharist, the Christ-bread whom Symeon holds, embraces, eats, and possesses in his heart. His mystical experience of the liturgy and the Bible makes him conscious that he is doing "in truth" what had been accomplished in history from the beginning of the world.

Then he saw the end: "I saw the life to come, untouched by corruption, which is Christ's gift to those who seek him, the kingdom of heaven already within me, where I found the Father, the Son, and the Spirit, three Persons of one undivided Godhead."

Symeon is united to the three divine Persons, who, together with human persons, act out history. Consequently, he is united mystically to all those who played some role in Bible history. He is Adam in the garden; he is Moses on the mount, kneeling unshod in adoration before the bush of fire; he is the entire people, victorious in their flight from Pharaoh. He is even the bitter lake in the desert, whose waters are miraculously sweetened by the healing wood, an image of the cross. He is Mary of Nazareth, who hears from the angel that she is to become the Mother of God. At the same time, he is the cripple at the pool and the man born blind and finally Lazarus, the beloved friend whom the Lord raised from the tomb.

Jesus is the chief actor in this drama of history, and it is with him above all that Symeon is united. Symeon confesses Christ's greatness and his own unworthiness and gives vent to the emotion that dominates his celebration of the Eucharist: wonder.

Symeon is in awe at what he has become by entering sacramentally and mystically into Christ's paschal mystery: temple of God, urn of manna, lamp, jewel-case, field of treasure, fountain, paradise, tree of life. All this is present in Symeon's "earthly and material essence," in his body, where God kindles the flame of love, the fire that blazes up "to the third heaven."

Symeon tells his monks that it is only by this experience that we can truthfully sing the words of the Easter chant, "We have seen the resurrection." Christ's resurrection is ours; the historical event is mystically repeatable. What Christ accomplished once for all in his own flesh, on the stage of history, he also accomplishes in our flesh. He is buried in our bodies and rises in our spirits. He who is eternally glorified, glorifies our humanity together with his.

---

1 *Yogaś-citta-vṛtti-nirodha.* Translating *citta* as 'heart' is not my idea; it is the preferred rendering of Swami Śri Yukteśwar and several other commentators.

2 Cf. Abhinavagupta, *Tantrāloka* 5 (pp. 189-207); *Tantrasāra* 5 (pp. 127-135).

3 1,12 (Gnoli, *Testi*, p. 38).

4 My favorite definition of chastity is 'Living one's sexuality in accordance with the Golden Rule'. For my part, in the spirit of devotional Christianity, I have entrusted my sex life as a celibate monastic to the Mother of Jesus, and she has never failed me.

5 Cf. *Mahānirvāṇa Tantra* 2,14-26 (pp. 16-18); 3,146-150 (p. 44); 4, 79-80 (pp. 55-56); 10,110-111 (p. 249).

6 Cf. Eliade, *Yoga* pp. 111-114; 261-267; 283-284.

7 *Vijñānabhairava Tantra* 142-145 (pp. 164-165).

8 Cf. *Śiva Sūtras* 3,27 (p. 46).

9 *Vijñānabhairava Tantra* 147 (p. 165).

10 Ibid., 149.

11 Ibid., 150-151 (p. 167).

12 Cf. idem, 155-162 (pp. 170-172).

Epilogue

The Yoga of Jesus

A New Testament text, Ephesians 3:17-19, gives us a prayer of the apostle Paul for his fellow disciples:

"May Christ dwell in your hearts through faith, and may love be the root and foundation of your life. Thus you will be able to grasp fully, with all the holy ones, the breadth and length and height and depth of Christ's love, and experience this love, which surpasses all knowledge, so that you may attain to the fullness of God."

We do not know whether Paul was thinking of the cross in speaking of these four dimensions, but there are abundant witnesses to this interpretation in ancient tradition. From earliest times, the cross of Christ has been seen as the link between different levels of reality: the invisible and inaccessible Godhead, the material cosmos in which the transcendent God is also immanent, and the in-gathering of the peoples of the earth into God's kingdom.

The cross is the key to the unity of cosmos and community. In the *Orthros* of Easter (the all-night paschal vigil of the Orthodox liturgy), the sepulcher of Christ is praised as the fixed point at the center of a turning world; from this center springs forth the 'new wine', the drink of immortality in the kingdom of God. The faithful sacramentally place themselves at this point, where they are buried and made to rise again with the Lord.

The cosmic extension is also expressed in the affirmation that the entire universe is the body of Christ. This is more than a mere metaphor, a figure of speech that makes no claim to reality. Paul and an important current of early Christian tradition see a real, ontological influence of Christ's humanity on the physical universe. The Word was made flesh, and this was possible because matter and human nature have an ontological openness to be taken up into the divine nature.

The redemptive work of Jesus on earth, in transforming humanity, transforms the entire universe, with which human existence and human fulfillment are bound up. We are not freed 'from' the world; we are simply made free, and the whole world is taken up into our freedom. The material universe "groans in the pangs of childbirth, as it awaits the revelation of the children of God" (Romans 8:19-23), because God's children already, here and now, enjoy the first fruits of the Spirit.

Here we find the heart of the yoga of Jesus: the cosmic dimensions of the cross. His self-offering for all humankind is the archetypal sacrifice, and his passage from death to life is his 'baptism', the archetypal initiation in which all are called to share. The nails that fixed Jesus to the wood immobilized him in the *āsana* that reflects the world-*maṇḍala*. The cross is his open-armed embrace of the world and all humanity, an embrace that heals all enmity and division. His last breath, with which he began the new age of the Spirit, is a true breath-sacrifice, a unique *prāṇāyāma* that has devoured time once for all and has freed us from its inexorable cycles. The cross of Jesus is above all the bejeweled cross of the resurrection, symbol of victory and freedom. Risen from the dead, the body of Jesus is now the mystical universe in which the fire of the Spirit descends from the Father, touches the earth with flame, and ascends again.

"With Christ I am nailed to the cross" (Galatians 2:19). I am a yogi by sharing in the yoga of Jesus, by participating in the mysteries of his life, death, and resurrection, but also by practicing the fire-rite of the tantric yogis, that of the breath offered to breath and so to God.

Let me share with you a final *kriyā* by which you can be where Jesus was, between his Mother and his beloved disciple on Calvary. Sit straight on your chair or meditation cushion. Place your hands on your breast and begin the *yajña* practice: Breathe in deeply and slowly through your nose and slightly-parted and relaxed lips, making with the breath the unvoiced vowel sound *ə* ('a' as in 'was'); having filled your lungs and without holding, breathe out with the same slowness, through nose and lips, forming with your mouth and tongue the unvoiced vowel-sound *i* (as in 'is'). If you ever need to swallow your saliva, do so when the breath is completely out, and then begin breathing immediately. Continue without interruption and repeat at least three times.

Then breathe in as before while extending your arms laterally from the shoulders, palms open and facing forward, as if you were on the cross. When your lungs are full, drop your head toward your right shoulder and breathe out slowly, making the breath-sound. (Jesus says to his mother, "Behold your son" [John 19:26].) When the lungs are empty, straighten your head, immediately breathe in as before, keeping the arms stretched out, and when the lungs are full, drop your head toward your left shoulder and breathe out slowly with the sound. (Jesus says to his disciple, "Behold your mother" [John 19:27].)

Finally, breathe in slowly with the unvoiced sound, and when your lungs are full, drop your head forward to your chest and breathe out. (Jesus breathed his last and gave over the Spirit [John 19:30].) When the lungs are empty, raise your head and begin breathing normally, with the mental *haṁ-saḥ* (lips closed). Lift your arms straight up and join the palms above your head, as if greeting God; then slowly lower them and hold the joined palms before your face, as if greeting a teacher; at last lower them to your breast, as a greeting to a dear friend.

The Jesus Prayer

Jesus is your friend, the intimate friend of all; he is like us in all things but sin. He is God by eternal birth, but he was born of a woman as we all were; he breathed the same air we breathe and died as we shall all die. Say to him from your heart, "Jesus." The name is enough, but if you wish you may add another word or words. There is no need to synchronize these words with your breathing, because the breath always produces its own, natural *mantra*, the *haṁ-saḥ*. Among Christian mantras are the following:

The mantra of the Apocalypse (Revelation 22:20): "Maranatha, come, O Lord."

The mantra of Thomas (John 20:28): "Jesus, my Lord and my God."

The Good Friday chant: "Savior of the world, save us."

The prayer of the Russian pilgrim: "Lord Jesus, Son of God, have mercy on me, a sinner."

Appendix

Yoga, Tantrism, and Symeon the New Theologian: Selected Sources

Patañjali, *Yoga Sūtras*:

Yoga Philosophy of Patanjali (containing his yoga aphorisms with Vyasa's commentary in Sanskrit and a translation with annotations including many suggestions for the practice of yoga), by Samkhya-yogacharya Swami Hariharananda Aranya, rendered into English by P. N. Mukerji (Albany, NY: SUNY Press, 1983).

Abhinavagupta (Kashmir, mid-tenth to early eleventh century):

Hymns. Translated by Lilian Silburn, *Hymnes de Abhinavagupta* (Paris: Boccard, 1970).

Paramārthasāra, translated by Lilian Silburn, *Le Paramārthasāra* (Paris: Boccard, 1958).

Tantrāloka, translated by Raniero Gnoli, *Luce delle Sacre Scritture (Tantrāloka) di Abhinavagupta* (Turin: UTET, 1972).

Tantrasāra, translated by Raniero Gnoli, *Abhinavagupta: Essenza dei Tantra (Tantrasāra)* (Turin: Boringhieri, 1960); chapters 1-3 translated by José Pereira, *Hindu Theology: A Reader* (New York: Doubleday Image, 1976), pp. 372-378.

Others of Abhinavagupta's School:

Kshemaraja, *Pratyabhijñahṛdayam*, translated by Kurt F. Leidecker, *The Secret of Recognition* (Madras: Adyar Library, 1938).

Maheshvarananda, *Mahārthamañjarī*, translated by Pereira, op. cit., pp. 381-388, and by Silburn (Paris: Boccard, 1968).

Vasugupta, *Śiva Sūtras*, ranslated by Pereira, op. cit., pp. 360-364; with the commentary by Kshemraja, translated by Jaideva Singh (Delhi: Motilala-Banarsidass, 1979).

Hindu Tantric Texts:

Mahānirvāṇa Tantra, translated by Arthur Avalon [John Woodroffe], *Tantra of the Great Liberation* (New York: Dover, 1972).

Mālinivijaya Tantra, translated by Gnoli, *Luce delle Sacre Scritture*, chapters 1-10.

Vijñānabhairava Tantra, translated by Lilian Silburn, *Le Vijñāna Bhairava* (Paris: Boccard, 1961).

Various texts related to Abhinavagupta's school:

Raniero Gnoli, translated, *Testi dello Sivaismo* (Turin: Boringhieri, 1962), including *Pāśupata Sūtras*, *Śiva Sūtras*, and *Spanda Kārikā*.

Buddhist Tantric Texts:

Śri-cakra-sambhāra Tantra, translated by Kazi Dawa-Samdup (London: Luzac: 1919).

Garma C. C. Chang, translated, *The Hundred Thousand Songs of Milarepa* (New York: Harper Colophon, 1970).

Chang, *Teachings of Tibetan Yoga* (Secaucus NJ: Citadel, 1974).

W. Y. Evans-Wentz, edited, *The Tibetan Book of the Great Liberation* (London: Oxford U. Press, 1972).

Evans-Wentz, *Tibetan Yoga and Secret Doctrines* (London: Oxford U. Press, 1967).

Evans-Wentz, *Tibet's Great Yogi Milarepa: A Biography from the Tibetan* (London: Oxford U. Press, 1972).

Herbert V. Guenther, translated, *The Jewel Ornament of Liberation by sGamPoPa* (Berkeley CA: Shambhala, 1971).

Guenther, *The Life and Teachings of Naropa* (London: Oxford U. Press, 1974).

Yoga and Tantrism, Secondary Sources:

Lama Anagarika Govinda, *Foundations of Tibetan Mysticism* (New York: Samuel Weiser, 1974).

Guenther, *The Tantric View of Life* (Boulder CO: Shambhala, 1976).

Silburn, *Kundalini: The Energy of the Depths: A Comprehensive Study Based on the Scriptures of Nondualistic Kasmir Saivism* (Albany NY: SUNY Press, 1988).

Symeon the New Theologian, Primary Sources (Greek text and French Translations):

Sources Chrétiennes (abbreviated 'S.C.'), various volumes and dates (Paris: Cerf).

Catéchèses [Catechetical Sermons or Discourses, abbrev. CT], edited by B. Krivochéine, Sermons 1-5 (S.C. volume 96, 1963); 6-22 (S.C. 104, 1964); 23-34 (S.C. 113, 1965).

Eucharisties [Thanksgivings, abbrev. EU], ed. by B. Krivochéine, 1-2 (S.C. 113, 1965).

Chapitres Théologiques, Gnostiques et Pratiques [Theological, Gnostic, and Practical Chapters, abbrev. TGP], ed. by J. Darrouzès (S.C. 51, 1957).

Traités Théologiques [Theological Treatises, abbrev. TT], ed. by J. Darrouzès (S.C. 122, 1966).

Traités Ethiques [Ethical Treatises, abbrev. TE], ed. by J. Darrouzès, 1-3 (S.C. 122, 1966); 4-15 (S.C. 129, 1967).

Hymnes [Hymns, abbrev. H], ed. by J. Koder, 1-15 (S.C. 156, 1969); 16-40 (S.C. 174, 1971); 41-58 (S.C. 196, 1973).

Symeon and Hesychasm, Secondary Sources:

George Maloney, *The Mystic of Fire and Light: St. Symeon the New Theologian* (Denville NJ: Dimension Books, 1975).

B. Krivochéine, *In the Light of Christ: Saint Symeon the New Theologian (949-1022), Life-Spirituality-Doctrine* (Crestwood NY: St. Vladimir's Seminary Press, 1986).

The Philokalia: The Complete Text, translated from the critical Greek editions by G. E. H. Palmer, Philip Sherrard, and Kallistos Ware (London: Faber and Faber, 1979 ff.).

Glossary of Terms and Index

experience, the direct, non-conceptual knowledge of a present reality: 4-9, 12-17, 22-29, 34-42, 47-59, 61-72, 75, 79-83, 87-92, 95-99, 103-104, 115, 117, 120-121, 123

eye: 28, 52, 54-56, 61, 63, 80, 82, 102-103

faith: 1-7, 12-17, 25, 38, 47-55, 62, 79-82, 89, 91, 97, 105. 111, 114, 117-119, 123

Father (God), the first Person (*hypostasis*) of the Trinity, together with the co-equal and eternal Son (or Word) and the Holy Spirit, whom Semitic Christianity (the church in India, Persia, Syria, and Lebanon) has always recognized as Mother (*ruh*, 'Spirit' in the Syriac language of their liturgy, being a feminine noun): 36, 47, 80, 106, 111, 120, 124

fathers (and mothers) of the church and the monastic order, early Christian teachers: 6-9, 48, 50, 80

fire, flame: 27-29, 32, 36, 47-48, 52, 61-70, 73, 79-83, 90, 95-107, 114-120, 124

flower, lotus, see 'plants'

flesh, see 'body'

focusing, *ekāgratā* (Sanskrit, 'one-pointedness'): 21, 28, 31, 34, 39, 62, 66, 72, 81, 85, 87, 89-91, 96-97, 103-104, 113

forehead: 28, 105, 116

fourth, according to the Indian scheme of 'the three and the fourth', in which three terms, in an immanent dialectic, are transcended by a fourth term (contrast with Western bipolar dialectics): 37, 85-87

freedom (see also '*jīvanmukta*', 'liberation'): 10, 19, 21, 23, 26, 33, 37, 41-42, 52, 55-58, 63, 69, 73, 85-86, 99, 102, 104, 110, 124

glory: 47, 51 53-56, 82, 101-104, 119

gnōsis (Greek 'knowledge' q.v.): 88

Gods: 30, 35, 68, 116-117

Gospel: 7, 57, 81, 117

grace: 12-15, 25, 37, 47, 53-57, 72, 75, 80-92, 95-107, 109, 117-121

gross, paired with 'subtle' (q.v.), refers more to the way of knowing than to the reality known: 22-23, 28-29, 33-34, 116

guru (Sanskrit 'authority', hence 'teacher', literally 'one who has weight, whose judgment is weighty'; according to folk etymology, 'one who leads us from darkness into light'): 1, 3, 17, 23-24, 33, 47, 62-63, 79, 83, 103, 105

haṁ-saḥ, the 'lesser *kriyā*' and the natural *mantra* of breathing, described in the *Vijñānabhairava Tantra* and in other yogic texts: 41-42, 66-67, 97-98, 115, 125

haṭha yoga is a physical discipline (postures and gestures, bodily hygiene, breath exercises) preparatory to meditation and the awakening of *kuṇḍalinī*: 27, 113

head, brain: 10-11, 27-28, 33, 36, 39, 52-53, 64, 66, 71, 103, 119, 125

heart center: 22, 27-30, 36, 39, 52, 55, 61-65, 71-74, 79, 81-86, 89, 97-98, 103-107, 109, 118-121, 123-126

heat, warmth: 52, 64-67, 84, 103

heaven, sky: 31, 51-55, 62, 65, 68, 73-74, 82, 87, 117, 119-120

Hesychasm, from the Greek word *hēsychia*, meaning 'quiet' or 'the silent life', is a spiritual path (also called 'the Jesus Prayer tradition') closely identified with the Eastern Church, developed and refined both as a way of life and as theology in monastic centers of the Mediterranean and Eastern Europe: 5-9, 47

Hinduism, a generic term for the spiritual traditions of India, which, although never dogmatically defined nor transmitted through hierarchical structures, have nonetheless preserved both a profound unity and a rich pluralism in doctrine, discipline, and devotional practice: 1, 5-6, 9-11, 17, 19-27, 31-32, 35, 48-49, 66-67, 70, 75, 83, 91, 97, 110, 113, 116, 119

history: 6-7, 12, 16-25, 47, 49-50, 70, 81, 114, 117, 119-121

icon (see also '*maṇḍala*'): 15, 23, 34-36, 109, 116

iḍā, see '*nāḍīs*'

image and likeness of God: 17, 58, 79, 81, 86-90, 99, 102

imagine, imagination: 14, 28, 69, 79, 89, 114

immortality (see also 'eternity', 'resurrection'): 21, 123

kriyā, ritual action, the act of sacrifice (*yajña*, q.v.), in the *YS* 2,1 the total practice of yoga embracing the last three *niyama* (q.v.), and in the teaching of Yogananda a yoga that awakens *kuṇḍalinī* and leads to cosmic consciousness or 'Christ consciousness': 1, 4, 12, 23, 27, 31, 36, 41, 66, 83-84, 103, 110, 112-113, 118, 124

kumbhaka, Sanskrit, meaning 'suspension' of breathing by holding the breath as if in a 'pot' (*kumbha*): 38

kuṇḍalinī, Sanskrit, meaning 'coiled' or 'serpentine', is the form of *śakti* (q.v.) residing in the human body as a potential force 'coiled' like a serpent at the base of the body's vertical axis, to be awakened by the practice of yoga, meditation, and/or religious devotion (see 'love'): 10, 21, 27-29, 33, 35, 39, 42, 47, 71, 96-97, 101, 114

law: 9-10, 19, 33, 69

liberation (see also 'freedom', '*jīvanmukta*'): 6, 22, 26, 32, 37-38, 52, 56, 63, 69, 86, 110, 115

life: 3-14, 26-27, 30-32. 47-53, 56-59, 61-64, 68, 80-92, 95-96, 100-107, 111-112, 115, 117-121, 123-124

light: 9, 37, 47-59, 61-73, 79-83, 87-92, 95-96, 102-106, 119-120

lightning: 10, 52, 53, 64, 104

liturgy: 7, 68, 117, 120, 123

love: 13, 15, 37, 56, 65, 68-75, 80, 83, 86, 96, 99, 102, 105-106, 109, 111, 115, 120, 123-126

maṇḍala, a sacred diagram, a symbolic temple, an initiatory ritual, and a support for meditation in tantric traditions, both Hindu and Buddhist: 34-36, 47, 116, 124

manifestation of God, of consciousness: 21, 28, 32, 36, 82, 86, 90, 96, 99, 101-103, 114

mantra (Sanskrit 'mental tool'), originally a mnemonic device used in memorizing the Vedas (q.v.), then an independent support for meditation by which the conceptual content of the word or words is transcended: 38-42, 47, 71, 87, 115-116, 125-126

marriage: 36, 61, 71, 73, 75, 83, 105-107

Mary, a virgin of Nazareth, who conceived by the Holy Spirit and gave birth to Jesus Christ, she is honored by the Church as the *The-*

consciousness transformed by faith and by the Holy Spirit dwelling within us: 1, 4, 6-9, 12, 14, 22, 29, 36, 47-59, 61, 65, 67-68, 72-75, 80-83, 89-92, 95, 98-99, 102, 105, 117, 120

nāḍīs (Sanskrit, 'channels') through which *prāṇa* (q.v.) flows in the body, especially *iḍā* and *piṅgalā*, entwined around *suṣumnā nāḍī*, the pathway of awakened *kuṇḍalinī* (q.v.) along the vertical axis of the body: 27, 31, 63, 66, 98

nature, divine: 7, 13-14, 29, 32, 47, 51, 57-58, 66-67, 70, 81, 83, 88, 95, 98-104, 124

nature, human: 5, 7, 12-13, 16, 25-26, 29, 32, 47, 51, 53, 57, 66, 72-73, 81, 83, 85, 88, 90-91, 95, 98-101, 106, 109, 118, 124

nirvāṇa (Sanskrit, 'cooling' of a fever, 'quenching' of thirst, 'blowing out' of a flame) is the supreme state in Buddhism and Hinduism, while in the tantric traditions it is usually paired with *saṁsāra* ('flowing-with' the current of causality) in the affirmation that the ultimate experience is that of *nirvāṇa* within *saṁsāra*, that is, of liberation within the flesh, the world, and time: 2, 28, 32, 83

niyama (Sanskrit, 'precepts' or 'observances'), five ascetical rules in the *YS* 2,32, named as 'cleanliness', 'contentment', 'fervor', 'study', 'surrender to the Lord', the last three of which are collectively called *kriyā-yoga* in *YS* 2,1 (see also *yama*): 23, 110, 112

objective salvation: 54

Orthodoxy, Eastern, see 'Eastern Church', 'Christianity'

Palamas, Gregory, fourteenth-century monk and theologian, great teacher of Hesychasm (q.v.), who elaborated a doctrine of the divine energies on the basis of his own and others' experience in the practice of the Jesus Prayer (q.v.): 8, 47

participation: 13-15, 62, 79, 87, 99-101, 117-118

particular means (see also 'divine means', 'energic means'): 37, 86, 103, 110, 113-117

passionlessness (translates Greek term *apatheia*), freedom from passions (q.v.), perhaps better understood as the restoration of integrity to our broken humanity and the progressive transformation of human life by grace: 69, 96